$19.95 (US)

Sex, Drugs & Rock N Roll
3 Keys For A Healthier Lifestyle

Dr. Nick Caras
Angel Tuccy

The information contained in this book is based on the personal and professional experience of the authors, and by no means intended to be a substitute for consulting your physician or health care provider. The authors do not dispense any medical advice or prescribe the use of any technique or treatment for any medical problems without the direct advice of a physician.

The authors and publisher specifically disclaim all responsibility for any liability or risk, which is incurred as a consequence of the use and application of the contents of this book.

If you cannot agree with the above statement, please put down this book and do not read any further. Your continued reading is your acknowledgement and agreement to hold harmless everyone connected with the production of this book.

3 Keys To A Healthier Lifestyle

Sex
More Sex & Intimacy

Drugs
Healthy Supplements & Nutrition

Rock N Roll
Fun Physical Activity & Exercise

Also by Dr. Nick Caras

Detoxify Your Lifestyle

Also by Angel Tuccy

Lists That Saved My Life

Lists That Saved My Business

Dedication

By Nick

To my amazing wife, for joining me on this crazy journey to

health and longevity.

I cannot wait to get to 100 years old with you.

By Angel

I dedicate this book to my family

for being my testing ground. I am so grateful for what we've

created as a family. Here's to family!

Sex, Drugs & Rock N Roll
3 Keys For A Healthier Lifestyle

Sex, Drugs & Rock N Roll
3 Keys For A Healthier Lifestyle

Table of Contents

Testimonials   *1*
Foreword   *3*
Preface   *9*

Chapter 1   *13*
America's Health Care Crisis

Chapter 2   *23*
Live Your Healthiest Life

Chapter 3   *29*
History Of Bad Drugs

Chapter 4   *35*
5 Stages Of Change

Chapter 5   *57*
More Sex

Chapter 6   *65*
Healthy Drugs

Chapter 7   *77*
Healthy Eating

Chapter 8
Make Time For Dinner   *91*

Chapter 9
Meal Planning   *99*

Chapter 10
Reading Your Blood Work   *111*

Chapter 11
Balanced Exercise Routines   *119*

Chapter 12
No More Excuses   *135*

Chapter 13
A Balanced Structure   *149*

Chapter 14
Super Recipes   *157*

Chapter 15
Checklists   *171*

Chapter 16
Plan For Success   *175*

Chapter 17
Resources   *179*

About The Authors   *187*

Testimonials

Dr. Caras simplifies and puts into words what our healthcare and educational system cannot. This book makes it easy for the average American to understand how to make their life healthier and happier for the long haul. - B.M.

I found this book to be an easy read. Dr. Nick gets to the point in simple terms that anyone can understand. This book is a good beginning to a healthy lifestyle. - J.O.

For me, I don't think there could be a better time than right now for setting goals and resolving to be better in so many areas of our lives. Angel's writing style is very conversational and I really felt like she could have been sitting across a table in a coffee shop telling me these stories and sharing her life. - M.C.

This book will teach you new things and hit you over the head with some old things that over time we all forget. You will find this book to be very conversational. Angel speaks right to you and provides tons of amazing insight. - L.H.

Foreword

Has anyone else noticed that our world and our lives are crazy?! Has technology helped us, or added more to our chaos? Is health care really any more advanced – or are we still sick and tired of being sick and tired?

These are just some of the typical questions I ask myself, and have asked patients and clients over all the years.

Let me give you some background – I too am a Mom, Chiropractor, Coach and Entrepreneur. My family lives the same full and busy life that you do. We are juggling schedules of three sons, both my husband's and my offices and careers, and also trying to coordinate food and home routines.

I've constantly asked, "Where are the common sense rules or guide for living?" Well, you hold that in your hands right now.

Authors Angel Tuccy and Dr. Nick Caras have laid out those notes or guides to those typical questions we all have.

In this book the authors have outlined why it's important for us to look at taking responsibility for our own health and well-being. As a society we have more knowledge and more technology in the health arena that ever before, yet why are we as a nation still sick? Why do we have major health issues either for ourselves, our family or friends?

We have a great health system for handling the crisis. If you think about a health issue like a fire, our system if fabulous for putting out the fire, dealing with the crisis. The challenge is what do you do to recover from that fire or crisis? And an even more powerful question is how do we prevent the problems and issues from arising? With our health care if we keep handling the things the way they have always been done, asking and answering the same questions, we will keep getting the same

4

results.

The book you hold in your hands will offer you a new paradigm, a new way of taking a look at your health and wellness. The authors show you why it's incredibly important to empower yourself, and to make wiser health choices and decisions for the next generation.

Once we are presented with how important it is to make new and empowered decisions for you and your family, then what? They provide an entire chapter on how to change and begin to create a new lifestyle and health habit pattern. As a coach I can reinforce the value and importance of learning these steps of change. Most people stay the same because it's too overwhelming to figure out how to get a new reality, end up in a different place.

The authors offer you insights on how to take the next simplest step on your journey. One step at a time you can shift, creating new health choices and patterns. Then the momentum begins to build. Once change leads to the next, and before you know if you have a new plan in place. Angel and Dr. Nick help guide you through this creation of a new plan, and the implementation steps.

You will be guided through decisions on everything from diet, nutrition, exercise, time management, meal planning, and raising healthy children.

You hold in your hands the first step and stage of creating a new reality for yourself, your family and your friends. Begin this journey with confidence; knowing it's the right and important next step. Each subsequent step and change along this path will enhance your health and wellbeing. Together the steps will build momentum. Within weeks and months you will become the new YOU, the person that you know you are destined to be!

To your health,

Dr. Janice Hughes

www.2inspireonline.com

Preface

Premier Chiropractic and Natural Medicine has become the go-to place for soccer moms in the suburb of Highlands Ranch, CO; not just for their chiropractic adjustments, but also for guidance on how to provide a healthier lifestyle for their family. Dr. Nick Caras and his team are in the business of bringing healthy back and eliminating the health care crisis that is consuming the American family. However, the biggest obstacle in creating a healthier lifestyle is the issue of time. As the pressure increases for moms to do more with less, the quick and modern conveniences have become mom's fallback plan to health. More and more, nutrition is being put on the back burner and family time at the dinner table is being sacrificed. Dinner in the drive-thru is picking up the slack and cardio workouts are limited to the dash from the house to the minivan. Rather than crunching abs, moms are left crunching more into their to-do list.

Sex, drugs and rock n roll is quickly becoming the new mantra for moms. What was originally the song of partying in Hollywood is now the cry of the suburban housewife. Your sex-drive isn't gone, but it's definitely seen brighter days. No longer are you looking for experimental party drugs to keep you revved up; instead, you're looking for healthy nutrition for your family and you need answers you can trust when choosing nutritional supplements. The rock-n-roll days of your youth are now being re-liberated as women all across the country discover that their unfulfilled dreams aren't dead, they are just waiting to be revitalized with new passion.

As a full-time working mom and business owner, Angel Tuccy struggles to be all things to her family and to her career as an author and talk show host. Angel's book, *Lists That Saved My Life,* became an instant hit among working mothers looking to bring more balance into their lives. In the constant pursuit of balance, it seems as if "health" is the easiest thing to put off until tomorrow. Well, tomorrow is finally here.

Today is the day to bring back more sex and intimacy into your relationships. Today is the day to dump the junk food and put your family on the path to health and wellness. Today is the day to pull out your dancing shoes, turn on the radio and rock n roll your way to happiness. Today is the day you take your family on a sprint toward health.

Chapter 1

America's Health Care Crisis

The health of America is in jeopardy. When Dr. Nick published his book, *Detoxify Your Lifestyle* in 2008, he hoped it would plant the seed for the health of our nation to improve. Even though he saw incredible desire for creating a healthier lifestyle, simply knowing the facts didn't create the permanent change readers were looking for.

Despite advancements in healthcare and pharmaceuticals, America is far from being the healthiest nation in the world. All the resources exist, yet we are much closer to being the least healthy.

If you are a fan of *Detoxify Your Lifestyle*, congratulations for changing your lifestyle and choosing to eat organic foods, exercising regularly, and pursuing a fulfilling lifestyle that helps our nation become a little bit healthier each day.

Every resource known to man is available to be able to live long, healthy lives. So, the question remains: why is there a health care crisis? Why are cancer, heart disease, and diabetes running rampant through our great country? There is an overwhelming majority of people who are unhappy with their lives, unfulfilled in their jobs, and disappointed with their family life. They have no energy and they feel run-down. Many resent their spouse. This is not the way life is supposed to be.

These are all issues that need to be addressed in the short years to come in order to turn the diseased state of our nation around. It is going to take an individual effort from each person to make a conscious effort to change.

If you were to pull out your fantasy mirror, you could imagine a lifestyle where you wake up excited about your day, filled with energy and ready to take on the needs of your family. Your day is full, but energizing. At the same time, you can't wait see your spouse and you enjoy family time each evening. The joy that life should bring you should be full of motivation and enthusiasism about each day. We want you to know right now that this is the way your life can be; and this book is going to show you how!

It's time to put sickness on the back shelf and regain the health of your family. They deserve it. You deserve it. Just think about the legacy that will be.

Bringing Healthy Back

It's time to bring "healthy" back. This book is written to help you get more out of your life; to be happier, more productive, and enjoy your life to the fullest.

The desire of your heart is to stop feeling tired. You want to be a role model for your family's health. You want more intimacy and you want to live a fulfilled life, not just a busy one. The problem isn't that you don't know what to do; you just need a little guidance and direction to get there. You will be able to use this book as a tool to help you plan a balanced, healthy, and enjoyable life.

Most likely, your life is not in total shambles. Even though you are not getting 100% enjoyment and fulfillment out of life, you think to yourself, "It's not that bad. It could be worse."

Or maybe it is. Maybe you feel as if your life is a total wreck; dealing with depression, anxiety, diabetes, fibromyalgia or a plethora of other "Lifestyle Diseases".

Most "Lifestyle Diseases" do not pose a threat to your immediate future but they are essentially killing you slowly and removing decades from your life.

Lifestyle Diseases

Everyone these days is connected to someone who has battled cancer, or has some form of heart disease such as high blood pressure or cholesterol problems. With diabetes being diagnosed in record numbers, you can't help but be affected. "Lifestyle Diseases" include obesity, daily headaches, eating disorders, addiction to painkillers or over-the-counter drugs, and chronic back and neck pain.

Can life really be enjoyed to the fullest with one or more of these conditions hindering you day in and day out? "Lifestyle Diseases" are not only creating a healthcare crisis in America, they are robbing you of precious time with your family.

"Lifestyle diseases are robbing you of precious time with your family."

Quality Of Life

The economic experts are warning that you are going to need a quarter to a half million dollars to pay for your medical coverage in retirement. Because of your medical care needs, it's estimated that your final ten years will be the most expensive decade of your life. There are a couple reasons behind this. First, due to advances in medical care, people are living longer. Secondly, this coverage is not going to be cheap, whatsoever. Don't be confused and think that just because you are living longer that you are going to be healthy. It used to be that people dreamed of living to the age of 100, with the assumption that you would still be contributing to society.

Now, living longer is not the goal, especially if it means living your last years in a hospital bed or taking handfuls of pain medication every few hours. The new mile marker is to have quality of life. It's time to start pursuing a *quality of life* and enjoying your life to the fullest. You are not merely meant to live long, but to live well.

A full and vibrant life is not meant to be a memory of your youth. Just because you are all grown up with children doesn't mean that you can't be fun to be around. Children laugh hundreds of times per day, and they want you to laugh with them. It's hard to laugh when you are in pain, but laughter is truly the best medicine. The next time your child finds something funny, search down in your belly and bring out your

19

laughter. People who laugh are full of life. Finding reasons to laugh is a great step towards a vibrant lifestyle.

"People who laugh are full of life."

"Lifestyle Diseases" steal your laughter. Have you noticed how grumpy people in their 70's, 80's and 90's seem to be? It doesn't have to be that way. You can still be thriving and enjoying life at all of these ages.

In a recent television interview, a very spry 114-year old man living here in America, talked about the early 1900's, 1930's and other long-ago decades. He is a phenomenon. It's unusual for anyone to live that long in life and still be living a fulfilling life. Why can't everyone live this long and feel that great at 114 years old? With the sparkle in his eyes, and the spring still in his step, you would have sworn this guy was only seventy or eighty years old.

In fact, in Dr. Nick's practice, he sees forty and fifty year olds that are much more unhealthy than this 114-year old man. This man's advice to everyone was simple : eat less food and stay at an optimal weight. You do not need a Harvard medical degree to know this, yet America is probably the most obese country in the world. It's long overdue, but it's time for our doctors to be trained in how to talk to their patients about weight loss, nutrition, and lifestyle. You don't need to spend more time with your doctor; you need get to know your produce manager. America doesn't need a prescription. America needs healthy sex, drugs and rock n roll.

What are the keys to a long healthy life that you can enjoy well into your hundreds? The good news is it is actually fairly simple. The key points have to do with sex, drugs and rock n roll, or in other words, *an active lifestyle, proper nutrition and living a fulfilled life.* . The bad news is, it takes will power and dedication to get there.

Chapter 2

Live Your Healthiest Life

It's easy to agree that America definitely has a health care crisis. Insurance premiums are skyrocketing while quality of care is going down. More and more people are getting sick. Congress is debating on what to do and what the best plan is to tackle the health care crisis. You cannot watch the news anymore without hearing something tragic about the our "health care crisis."

New pharmaceuticals are hitting the market everyday as the "answer pill" to the most recent affliction of ailments. The disclaimers that come along with the new colored pill of the day are astronomical. Taking a pill for one symptom seems to bring on more issues to need a pill for. Now, instead of one pill, you end up taking three or four, and you still haven't cured anything. America doesn't need more pills; we need more healthy people.

Instead of piling on new band-aids, doesn't it make more sense to teach people how to be healthy? If more people were healthy, there would be no health care crisis. All of the major diseases from cancer, diabetes, heart disease, and obesity are all "Lifestyle Diseases" that can be prevented.

An Ounce Of Prevention

Prevention is a key to getting rid of the health care crisis. You would save literally thousands of dollars throughout your lifetime if you chose a preventative lifestyle and it would save our country billions of dollars as a whole. By living a wellness lifestyle and maintaining your health throughout every stage of life, you will obviously feel better and be more productive but there's more than that. You will drastically reduce the expenses associated with sickness and disease. You will be more energetic for your family. You will be able to pursue your passions and find purpose in your day.

Life expectancy keeps going up and will continue to go up. Over the past seventy years, life expectancy has gone up by about twenty years. This means if you were born in the 1970's, your life expectancy at that time was to live to about seventy years old. With the advancement of modern medicine, the fact is, now you will live much closer to the age of ninety.

Open The Photo Album

So, the question becomes, what would you like your life to be like when you reach 75, 85, 95 or even 100 years old and beyond?

One good trick to see what's coming down the health care path for you is to take a look at your parents, your grandparents and even your great-grandparents. What do they look like? How do they feel? How do they act? How are their energy levels? What about their posture? How is their skin? What about their attitude toward life? Are they stricken with diabetes, high cholesterol, blood pressure issues or Alzheimer's?

By taking a look at your older loved-ones, you have a sneak peak into what the future holds for you. Is it grim or exciting? Are you following in their footsteps because it's the only way you've ever known?

"Life expectancy has increased by 20 years."

You must understand that you do not suddenly get sick at the age of seventy years old. You have been working towards that sickness or disease for many decades. You don't suddenly have high cholesterol one day; it gradually increases over your lifetime. You don't get diabetes in one day; many years of unhealthy eating and lack of exercise builds up to diabetes. Cancer doesn't attack you in one particular day; it will grow slowly in an unhealthy body until one day you finally feel a symptom and head to the doctor's office. Pain is typically the final symptom that sends you to the doctor's office, but the symptoms have usually been there festering for ages.

Learn from those who have gone before you. You don't have to follow in the same sickly footsteps. Take a close look at your older generation and learn what they did wrong and why their quality of life is not the greatest. Your health history does not have to repeat itself.

On the other hand, healthy senior citizens have a lot to teach, too. Seek out older people who are not on any medications, who have great energy levels, and who are enjoying life to the fullest.

Learn from the feet of the masters of lifestyle. When you are eighty-five years old, wouldn't you love to be golfing, hiking, playing with your grandchildren or great-grandchildren, and still be productive in society? You were meant to have that quality of life and live the life of your dreams.

When it comes to establishing healthy habits for your family, don't let pharmaceutical advertisements be your guide. You need to be the one who teaches your family about the importance of eating well, managing stress and how to enjoy life. Your children will do what you do. Your good habits will become their good habits.

Chapter 3

A History Of Bad Drugs

A common trend in the medical field over the last five to eight years is that you don't have to be very old at all to be stricken with many serious medical conditions. There are many, many people who are still in the prime of their lives who have heart disease, who take several medications every single day, and have no energy. These are thirty-five to fifty year-old people who should be much better off at their age, but who have never been taught how to be healthy.

As children, you were brainwashed to think that a pill could fix everything. As soon as you had an earache as a child, your parents would run you up to the family doctor to get an antibiotic. As you got a little older, you would fall at the playground or get hurt playing sports and soon run back to the

29

doctor for a painkiller or anti-inflammatory pill. Throughout your teenage years, you would either have anxiety or depression; so back you went to the doctor for more medication. As you moved into your twenties and thirties, you were living in the real world, which meant headaches and high blood pressure. That's right, more pills and medications every morning. And now, that same legacy is being passed on to your own children.

In the last sixty years, American families have surrounded themselves with cheap, calorie-rich, nutrient-lacking foods, an increase in over-the-counter drugs and they have largely eliminated physical activity from their busy days. This is no way to live life to the fullest.

Recently, a thirty-one year old male walked into Dr. Nick's office for chronic neck and back pain. As they were going through his initial consultation and health history, Dr. Nick was beside himself when he read through his medication list. This healthy thirty-one year old was on every heart disease medication imaginable.

He'd had a heart attack and open-heart surgery at the very young age of twenty-nine. This was a first for Dr. Nick. He had never personally met someone who'd had a heart attack and open-heart surgery this young in life. Unfortunately, this is the trend we are starting to see with the lifestyle choices here in America.

"Your health is in your hands."

Start Today

The purpose of these stories is to make you concerned enough to look in the mirror and choose to make healthier changes starting today. By now, you realize that you don't live in the healthiest nation in the world, but there is good news. Your health is really in your hands. You get to make choices every single day about what to eat, how to properly exercise, and how to de-stress each night.

For starters, how about trading in your morning coffee and sugar for a *Green Drink*? A *Green Drink* is a mixture of twenty different vegetables in powder form that you combine with water or take in a capsule. Even if you're a fairly healthy individual today, you need to start thinking long-term about what you can improve on for the next few decades of life and how you can change your family's health legacy. Even your children can gulp down a *Green Drink* every morning to ward off the infestation of germs they are faced with every day at school. Even though you can't see it, your lifestyle is destroying your body from the inside out.

There is a better way of life than running to various doctor's appointments every month. Life is a long journey, and you want to be ready for it. As long as you keep climbing up, you will eventually reach the mountaintop. We want to help make sure you can still breathe and enjoy the view when you get there.

Angel's Secret To A Flat Tummy

If you have that roll of belly fat that no amount of exercise seems to get rid of, try a 3 – 10 day detoxifying cleanse. This is also great for that "after party" regret.

Drink *The Ultra Broth* for nutrition & cleansing
(recipe in back of book)

Drink plain green tea & water with lemon to quench thirst, detoxify and add antioxidants.

Each night, soak in a hot 20-minute bath with 1 cup of Epson salts for detoxifying. Add 7 drops of lavender for relaxing.

Start and end each day with 15 minutes of a cleansing yoga stretch.

Chapter 4
Stages Of Change

It takes forty-five days to change a habit or incorporate a new one. Most people in this day and age have many unhealthy and unproductive habits they perform on a day-to-day basis. These practices make you a little unhealthier each day, a little more unproductive each day, but yet you keep practicing these habits because they are just that – habits. You know you shouldn't be drinking that sugar-laden coffee each morning or you shouldn't be sleeping in when you could wake up and get a thirty-minute workout in before the day starts. You know the habits that you could and should change about your lifestyle, yet for whatever reason, you don't.

Most patients who come into see Dr. Nick rarely change their lifestyle in one single event. The patient moves gradually from being resistant or uninterested, to considering a change and then to finally deciding to go at the change 100% of the way. They may relapse on the way, but as long as they keep pushing forward, a new, healthier habit will finally form.

Change doesn't happen "cold turkey" all in one day. Although, under drastic circumstances, when it's brought on by a tragic situation, people can decide to change immediately and never look back, but it is definitely not the normal pattern. Behavioral change happens over time.

"Your lifestyle determines your health."

Dr. Nick had a terminally-ill cancer patient who quit his horrible lifestyle in one day when he made the internal decision that he didn't want to die; he wanted to live. He started eating nothing but fruits and vegetables. Immediately, he quit smoking, only drank water, and started on a very rigorous exercise routine, all in the same day he stepped foot into Dr. Nick's clinic for the very first time. It wasn't easy for him, but he made the decision in his head to just do it, and of course, he beat his cancer and is still very healthy today. He is a living, breathing testimony that your lifestyle determines your health.

The point is; do not wait for a very serious health risk or a life and death situation to persuade you to change your unhealthy habits. Start changing today and you can live a long, healthy life.

5 Stages Of Change:

1. Thought Stage – Thinking about changing a habit.

2. Effort Stage – Putting forth new choices.

3. Relapsing Stage - Slipping back into comfortable patterns.

4. Cycling Stage – Repeating the sequence.

5. New Lifestyle - Your new choices become part of your daily life.

When you follow the *5 Stages of Change*, you can create your own wellness lifestyle for you and your family.

Thought Stage

The *Thought Stage* is when someone is considering the pros and cons of developing a new habit. People will ponder change and then make excuses and reject it. This stage can last for months or even years as people know they want a better life for themselves and their family but are not willing to put forth the effort to change. How many times have you heard someone say they wanted to quit smoking, or they know they need to get that gym membership or start cooking dinner at home? You know someone who keeps saying they need to change but they just never get around to doing it.

At this stage of the game, you know change must occur, but you either don't have the willpower to go for it, or you might just be too lazy to get off the couch and do it.

During Dr. Nick's years of private practice, he's seen many young adults who know they should be leading a healthier lifestyle, but they are still in the habit of getting fast food on a daily basis because it seems so easy. Choosing to bring a healthier brown-bag lunch to work feels like it will be too much of a hassle.

More often than not, a mother of young children will complain that her children are sick all the time, or they feel tired and just can't seem to get on top of their health. Even though the answer is right in front of their nose, their patterns or habits keep them from making any permanent changes.

The pros have not outweighed the cons yet. Even though it's obvious where your life might be headed; years of high stress, high blood pressure, cholesterol issues, obesity, diabetes, or cancer are all waiting in line to get to your weakened immune system. But ultimately the choice is on you. You have to wake up one day and really decide for yourself to *change*. You will only move beyond this *Thought Stage* when you finally decide the positives outweigh the negatives. At this point you will then move into the *Effort Stage.*

Effort Stage

During the *Effort Stage,* you have actually made a bold commitment to change and you've put a lot of thought into changing your negative habit. Whether that habit is to quit smoking, start eating better, or start a new exercise routine, the pros have now outweighed the cons and you are ready to go for it. The *Effort Stage* is very exciting and your anticipation is high. Most likely, fear brought you here, and now, you're full of hope. The realization has sunk in that there are consequences if you keep to your old ways and those consequences scare you. Fear is one of the best motivating factors that will contribute to changing a habit, but *you don't have to wait for the fear factor.* You now have serious intention to change. You might not know how exactly to go about it, but you do know that you must start to move away from a habit that is affecting you negatively.

"Don't underestimate the power of your money."

You don't have to undertake this change all by yourself. You can always find someone to help you and support you, if you look for it. There are books, licensed professionals, support groups, and websites to help you on your journey to becoming healthier, more organized, and more productive in your life. Whether you are a Fortune 500 CEO or a stay-at-home mom, there is help for you. People who invest money in themselves have a much higher chance of succeeding with their lifestyle change.

Do not underestimate the power of your money. Once you spend money on a weight loss coach, you are more likely to lose weight and keep it off rather than if you tried to just lose weight on your own.

By investing in a coach, doctor, or a support group, you give yourself a much higher chance for success because you now have someone to keep you accountable to your new habit. The accountability factor is one that is often overlooked in success, but it is often where the most value is found. If you look at the most successful people in the world, they will have coaches and people that they look up to that keep them accountable. Hiring a coach almost guarantees you'll see quicker success because you're more likely to stay consistent and stick with it. Your coach won't let you fail. You may let yourself slip, but your coach won't and you'll be thankful for it.

During the *Effort Stage* you may still not trust that change is actually going to happen or that it is going to be permanent at this point. But you are at least giving it a shot. Sustaining the new habit is the real tough part in making any new lifestyle change. As humans, it is always easy to revert back to old habits; even though you know it is not the best decision. You must stay very strong during this stage of the game and it always helps to have support.

Stay surrounded by supportive friends, neighbors, and family when trying to get healthier. Hang out with people who are also motivated to live a healthy life. Choose to associate with dreamers and those who are excited about life.

Nothing makes us happier than when a whole family is turned onto a healthy lifestyle. Families that are eating right, exercising together, having great quality family time, and sleeping enough hours each night will be far less likely to attract the common cold, influenza, and even less likely to be on any medications. Choose not to be a statistic for the average family in America who is overmedicated and run down.

You can start the healthy revolution in your own family by making small changes that will bring you more energy, help you look better and feel better. It is amazing how the body responds to a great lifestyle. Your immune system will be much more effective, your blood pressure will stay at optimal levels, your energy levels will be high throughout the entire day and your overall satisfaction level with life will be great!

You need to remind yourself of these things when you are in the initial phase of the *Effort Stage*. You must constantly remind yourself of how great it is going to be once you get out of this rut.

"When you feel good, your sex life is revitalized."

The *Effort Stage* is really the basis of this book coming together. Dr. Nick has had hundreds of patients during his years of practicing natural medicine and chiropractic that get stuck in the *Effort Stage*. Initially, the staff at Premier Chiropractic is very good at motivating patients to put in the effort and make the initial change for a couple weeks. At about day 14-21, the results are showing and the patient feels great. They feel better than they've felt in a very long time, they are sleeping through the entire night, no longer need four cups of coffee to get them through their work day and, their sex life is revitalized because they finally feel good again. Life is now good, and then what happens? Little by little, they start to revert back to their old ways. One day, they think to themselves, "I am just going to skip my workout today, it

46

won't hurt anything." Or, "I might just have a fast-food cheeseburger and fries once this week for lunch. What can that hurt?"

Before you know it, they are completely back to their old habits. About three months later, they sluggishly come walking back into the clinic to ask what happened and why they feel run-down again. Well, it's not rocket science. They need a reminder and encouragement to reposition their thought process to get them back on the right track. This takes you to the next couple stages of change – *Relapsing and Cycling*.

Relapsing Stage

Do not be afraid of relapsing. Everyone has been there and it is part of the process. It is okay. Sometimes relapsing can actually be a positive thing. Relapsing can be an effective reminder that your nasty habit doesn't feel good and show you how badly it's taking its toll on your body and well-being.

47

Just as in the example above, someone can quit eating fast-food for a few weeks and start to look and feel great, but once they are back in their "supersized" drive-through lifestyle for a couple weeks, they are quickly back to feeling toxic. This is a typical scenario and it is even a natural progression that people must go through in order to make a permanent change.

A lot of research shows the tipping point for change to be 45-60 days. Once you have cut out a particular habit for this long, your chances of success go way up for never relapsing again. It is critical to maintain a very positive attitude and to have support to lean on until you get this far in the game.

We recommend you make 90 days your goal before you officially celebrate. Two to three months is a great benchmark for a lot of people, but relapsing can also occur at any time. Ninety days is a blip in time, but worth every new moment it will bring to you.

When you go through the initial health consultation at Dr. Nick's office, he always checks to see if the new patient is a smoker or not. Every single person that has checked "yes" on this question always has a story or an excuse about how he or she cannot quit smoking. They have all tried and failed.

"Research shows the tipping point for change is 45-60 days."

Smoking isn't the only area of relapse. We've seen this same scenario with patients who went to a vegan diet for years, but now are back to eating refined and fried foods and processed meats again.

It is always the same answer; one big stressful or even tragic event forced them into relapse. Events such as loss of a parent, loss of a job, a divorce, or financial crisis forced them instantly into relapse. We understand that there is no way of avoiding extremely stressful events throughout a lifetime. Let's face it; everyone is going to experience loss, job stress, financial worries and much, much more. There is just no way around it. You must be especially strong at these times and understand that reverting to an old nasty habit is not going to fix the problem at hand. Much to the contrary, reverting to bad habits will actually increase your stress levels and decrease your body's own natural defenses to deal with the stress.

Any type of stressful or tragic situation in our life will raise your blood pressure, decrease healthy sleep patterns and reduce your sex-drive. By adding in another preventable stress such as eating unhealthy fast food, drinking caffeine all day long or not exercising because you are feeling sorry for yourself will only add to your body's inability to be healthy. As a chiropractic physician, Dr. Nick knows and believes that your body is constantly striving to be healthy. You are meant to be healthy from the day you were born until the day you die. You can strive to help your body's innate ability to be healthy by continuing to add in healthy habits and quit unhealthy habits. You can prepare your body to deal with the stresses that life throws at you.

Remember that stressful situations are not going away anytime soon, especially here in America's fast-paced lifestyle. Binge eating due to stress is not the answer. If anything, you should be extra careful during stressful times and create even more healthy habits to help you through this time. Dr. Nick is constantly telling his patients to double up on their vitamins, fruits and vegetables during stressful times to give the body the extra boost that it needs during that temporary period. Unfortunately, most people revert to relapsing during the hardest periods of life. You must stay strong, find a shoulder to lean on, and keep pushing forward.

Cycling Stage

The *Cycling Stage* is just as it sounds. You will keep going back and forth until you reach the tipping point that allows you to never look back again. As we've mentioned before, research shows that anywhere between 2-3 months is the most common tipping point. If you are trying to cut your coffee habit, grab a calendar and mark sixty days out. Tell yourself that you will not have a cup of coffee until that day and then replace your coffee habit with a new, healthier drink of choice. To eliminate a bad habit, you must replace it with a healthier one.

If you can make it without even one cup of coffee to your goal day, chances are you will not want to drink coffee anymore. Your body won't even crave it. On your first try, it will probably be very hard to get to day sixty. It's a pretty lofty goal. You might make it one week, maybe ten days, and then your inner willpower may weaken and you will find yourself in the coffee drive-thru line. This is a natural part of the process.

Realize that tomorrow is a new day and you get to make another decision on what you want to choose that day. That is the great part about life. Tomorrow always comes. The choice is always yours whether you are going to change or stay with your old habit. If you are willing to change and willing to put in the work, you are going to eventually make it to day sixty, day ninety, day one hundred twenty, and your new change will be part of your healthy lifestyle at that point.

New Year's Resolutions

Do you know how long New Year's resolutions usually last? Until January 7th. One week. January is notorious for *Relapses and Cycling*. Ninety-nine percent of people can barely keep their New Year's resolution one week. This is because they never made it past the *Thought Stage*. Remember, changing a habit is a serious process and a serious decision. You cannot decide on December 31st that you are going to quit eating red-meat, and think that on January 1st everything is going to be good-to-go. You must go through all five steps; *Thought, Effort, Relapse, Cycling,* and then finally, *New Lifestyle.*

From a professional chiropractor's opinion, it doesn't matter how long someone cycles, as long as they have put in the thought, weighed the pros and cons, and are making a serious effort. Your chiropractor will be here to help as long as you are serious about changing.

The more people cycle, the more it tells us they need more professional help. This is the time to invest in *you* and get the experts working on your side. Though well meaning, sometimes a spouse, a family member, or a friend is just not enough. If you can't get past the hurdles on your own, seek the help of a licensed professional who is properly trained to help you make a lasting change. Once you invest in yourself, the relapsing and cycling period will be drastically reduced.

New Lifestyle

Okay, you've finally made it and you are never looking back. You made the change that you set out to make and it is now simply part of your lifestyle. You no longer have to battle your bad habit, as a matter of fact you don't even think about your bad habit anymore. Your new behavior or lifestyle change is now your routine. It has been anywhere from three to six months now, and you are feeling great. You are getting more done each day. You are not procrastinating anymore. You have much more energy, you're having more sex, and you have a renewed outlook on life. Life is exciting again, and you look forward to getting out of bed each day, taking life by the horns and succeeding in each and every endeavor you decide to tackle.

Keep Going

Now that you have changed one bad habit, why not go for more? It is important not to try to change too much at any given time. One habit at a time is great progress. Give yourself a chance to succeed. After you make one lifestyle change, you can then move on to the next bad habit and turn that into a positive lifestyle change. Remember, this life is a long one, and in a couple years from now, you can be one hundred times healthier, more vibrant, and more successful than you are right now. Throughout every stage of life, you must persist and keep working on yourself in order to be better in every aspect of your life.

Chapter 5
More Sex

Having sex is a fulfilling key to a healthy lifestyle. Yet, more and more often, sex gets put on the back burner because you are tired, overworked or in a state of pain. It's hard to feel joy when your body aches. It's even harder to make someone else feel good when you feel awful. Creating a healthy lifestyle is a key component to a healthy sex life.

Enjoying a better sex life is a discovery process. When you discover fun ways to say "yes", and bring more intimacy into your relationship, your immediate view on life improves. The world is already full of rejection; make sure your marriage bed isn't. When it comes to bringing the love back into a struggling relationship, start by regenerating your sex life.

Discover Your Mate

Touch each other even when you're away from the bedroom. Hold hands when you're out in public. Look your lover in the eyes and hold his gaze for just a moment too long. Shower together. Undress in front of each other. Put love-making back on your to-do list and watch your entire family culture improve.

Let Go

It's hard to be angry and love each other at the same time. Relationships are not fair and everything is not always equal. It's okay to let a few things slide once in a while. It's okay to overlook minor issues. Humanity is not perfect, nor would you want it to be. Accept the differences that you thought were adorable in the beginning but annoy you now. Choose to be happy in your relationship.

Beautiful Lovers

Put some effort into your appearance. When you take a few minutes to pamper yourself, you'll feel prettier – even beautiful.

Beautiful women make beautiful lovers, and all women are beautiful to their lovers. Wrinkles and cellulite soften in dim lighting, so turn down the lights and light some candles. Don't make love in the pitch dark; let your mate see you. He wants to see you.

When you're in the shower, take a few extra minutes and shave your legs. Unshaven legs are the number one killer in the romance department. Your lover probably says he doesn't care, but it will definitely impact how you feel about yourself and stubble greatly increases inhibition.

Brush your teeth. Run a brush through your silky hair. Put on a fresh outfit everyday. Sloppy clothes are okay once in a while, but let's not make that your regular fashion statement.

Staying hydrated keeps your skin, lips and bodily fluids moist, so make sure you drink plenty of water during the day. Practice your kegal exercises to increase blood flow to the pelvic area.

The Bedroom Is For Romance

When you're at a loss for which room of the house to clean up and organize, start with the bedroom. Make sure your bedroom speaks of love and romance. Give your room a romantic overhaul if it needs it. Remove pictures of the grandparents and children; it's not good feng shui for romance. Instead, add photos of the two of you while on vacation and expressing love for each other. Eliminate the millions of extra bed pillows and cute stuffed animals and it will be easier to make your bed every day.

Be Honest

Tell your husband he is a great lover. He needs to hear it straight from your lips. Whisper it in his ear. If you don't feel like he's a great lover, help him discover what makes your purr so that you can be honest with him. Honesty is the backbone to great love-making. Don't ever fake it. In an intimate relationship, faking it is just not necessary.

When you bring the sex back into your relationship, the loose pieces of the communication puzzle fall back into place and your entire family reaps the benefits.

To the Wives:

You are beautiful. To your husband, you are the most beautiful person in the world. All day long, advertisements and other women are visually stimulating your spouse, and yet he waits for you until the end of each day. Be there for him with shaved legs.

To the Husbands:

Listen to your wife. Stop everything and give her your undivided attention. Tell her how much you appreciate her. Take the time to discover what pleases her outside of the bedroom as well as inside.

Top 10 Benefits Of A
Healthy Sex Life

Releases Endorphins

Reduces Stress

Pillow Talk Improves Communication

Improves Your Relationship

Increases Self-Esteem

Burns Calories

Heightens Energy Levels

Boosts Your Immune System

Helps You Sleep Better

Gives You A Reason To Stay Home On Saturday Night

Your Husband's Top 10 Reasons
For Having Sex

Because I woke up

Because I just got home

Because we're in bed together

Because we're in the same room together

Because I like you

Because it's Sunday, Monday, Tuesday, Wednesday, Thursday, Friday, or Saturday

Because we have a (marriage) license

Because we're on vacation

Because we're not on vacation

Because we can

Chapter 6

Healthy Drugs

There are literally thousands of supplements, vitamins, minerals, and drinks on the market today. Even your local gas station claims to sell vitamins and these so-called vitamin energy drinks. You cannot watch the 5 o'clock news without hearing about some new vitamin that will cure a specific disease. Proper vitamins and supplementation can help you beat most (if not all) diseases out there, but who do you believe and what should you really be taking? In reality, you could spend thousands of dollars a month on vitamins and still not be taking everything on the market today.

We are going to go through the *BIG 3* with you in this chapter. The *BIG 3* are what the average human body needs to be taking on a daily basis. These core supplements are for everyone –

kids, adults, black, white, healthy, or unhealthy, skinny, or obese. Everyone needs the *BIG 3*.

"Everyone needs the BIG 3"

Of course, there are supplements for virtually every single disease that could possibly walk into Dr. Nick's office, but the *BIG 3* vitamins/supplements we are going to explain for you in this chapter are the ones you should be taking for overall health, wellness, and longevity. It's important for you to seek professional advice if you are treating a specific illness.

Fish Oil

If there were just one supplement you could take daily for the rest of your life, it should be *Fish Oil*. The reason you need to take it is because fish oil contains an amazing nutrient called omega-*3* fatty acids (or omega 3's.) Do not confuse fish oil with other omegas such as omega-6 or omega-9 that you might be getting from flax oil or other supplements. It is very important to remember that your omegas need to come from fish oil such as salmon.

"Fish oil naturally lowers bad cholesterol."

The benefits of fish oil supplementation are endless. Number one – it helps prevent the two biggest killers in America today, which are heart disease and cancer. That should be reason enough. These two diseases account for a majority of the deaths in America, and by simply taking this supplement; you can really increase your odds of defeating these two nasty diseases. Fish oil defeats heart disease in a lot of different ways. It will naturally lower your blood pressure and bad cholesterol while raising your good cholesterol. It will also strengthen the inner lining of your arteries and it also has an anti-clotting effect on your arteries. Fish oil has also been shown to increase your chances of surviving a stroke or a heart attack. Right now, you should be thinking, "Here fishy, fishy. I need my fish oil."

Heart disease and cancer are not the only benefits of this super-supplement. It also is great on your brain and nervous system. The majority of your brain is made up of the essential omega 3 fats from fish oil. This is why your children most definitely need to be taking a fish oil supplementation. As the brain and nerves are developing early on in life, children will get the most benefit from supplementing with fish oil. This is especially important for children with neurological disorders such as ADD, ADHD, anxiety, and depression. A lot of times, fish oil can clear up these disorders on its own without any medications.

Fish oil is also great for your skin, nails and hair. Do you want to continue looking young and vibrant as you age? If the answer is yes, then fish oil supplementation is a must.

Probiotics

Most of the general public is very confused of what probiotics really are. In a nutshell, a probiotic supplement is a capsule of live bacteria. Do not get scared just yet. Bacteria are very, very important to your livelihood. They line and live in your intestines and digestive tract. They are very essential to life. There are actually more bacteria living inside your digestive tract than the number of cells in your entire body. That's a lot of bacteria.

There is a difference between good and bad bacteria. The bad bacteria cause infection and disease inside you while the good bacteria have many positive functions inside your body. These good bacteria in your digestive system actually make up more than 70% of your immune system. For you to be as strong and healthy as possible, your good bacteria need to be thriving on a daily basis. Unfortunately, most of us have wiped out our good bacteria population. Therefore, it needs to be replenished with probiotic supplementation.

The population of good bacteria gets wiped out in many different ways. First and foremost, every time throughout your life (or your child's life) that you have taken a round of antibiotics, it kills your good bacteria. Antibiotics are meant to kill bacteria (bad bacteria) when you get an infection. Guess what? The antibiotic does a great job of killing the bacterial infection thus getting you well, but in the meantime it has also killed all the good bacteria that are essential to life. After a round of antibiotics, your immune system is much weaker than before because, remember, most of your immune system lives within these good bacteria. This is why you see many kids getting bacterial infections over and over again. It is a very vicious cycle. The alternate solution is to strengthen your immune system rather than wipe it out. Daily probiotic supplementation will positively increase the strength of your immune system, thus decreasing the chances of ongoing bacterial infections. Doing it this way will also decrease your chances of getting many other diseases.

Probiotic supplementation is essential on a daily basis to keep your digestive tract and immune system working great. Examples of good bacteria are acidophilus, lactobacillus, and probulardi. We suggest getting a probiotic supplement that contains many different kinds of bacteria. You can also get good bacteria through a few food sources like yogurt, sauerkraut, and other fermented foods, but since most families don't eat a lot of these on a regular basis; your best bet is to take a probiotic every morning.

Green Drinks

We have mentioned *Green Drinks* throughout this book and by this time you're probably wondering what in the world is a *Green Drink*? A *Green Drink* as a vegetable and fruit supplement. We call it *Green* to overemphasize the importance of vegetables and their anti-cancer, anti-disease, and detoxifying affects they have on the human body.

The phytonutrients in a *Green Drink* are something you need every single day in order to fight off age-related diseases, fend off infections, and ensure you have an abundance of energy and vitality every day up to 100 years old and beyond. You can make your own *Green Drink* if you have a juicer or there are many drinks and powders on the market today as well. Juicing is a great way to get all your essential fruits and vegetables into your system on a daily basis, but for most people, it is much easier to put a scoop of a green powder supplement into a glass of water and get your *Green Drink* in that manner. *Green Drinks* can also come in capsule form. A *Green Drink* beverage a great breakfast option and a great way to start your day.

Let's face it; you are not serving your family over twenty servings of fruits and vegetables a day. Most of the *Green Drinks* on the market have over twenty servings of fruits and vegetables in them. This is a great way of satisfying your daily intake of fruits and vegetables in one simple drink. Don't make the mistake of thinking that by consuming a *Green Drink* in the morning that you can skip out on eating any fruits and vegetables during the day. Vegetables and fruit still need to be eaten. Think of your *Green Drink* as an insurance plan to make sure you and your family are getting enough vegetables every single day of your life. If your family is overtaken by the morning rush and tends to skip out on breakfast, you can take your *Green Drink* to go.

By taking a *Green Drink* every day, you will be getting the right nutrients to help detoxify the body each day ensuring a long, healthy life.

Some of the major ingredients to look for in a *Green Drink* include the following:

Wheat Grass	*Chlorella*	*Broccoli*
Alfalfa	*Spirulina*	*Cauliflower*
Carrot	*Coriander*	*Parsley*
Spinach	*Turmeric*	*Grapeseed*
Blueberries	*Pomegranate*	*Aloe Vera*
Green Tea	*Rosemary*	*Milk Thistle*

We know what you're thinking; "This is not going to taste very good." Dr. Nick has tasted many *Green Drinks* in his life. We will not lie to you, some of them do not taste the best, but there are several on the market that taste great. The fruit in most of the *Green Drinks* will give it a sweet taste and most of the high quality companies now add Stevia™ to their *Green Drinks*, which is an all-natural sweetener. Make sure you do not buy a green supplement that has added sugar or artificial sweeteners such as aspartame or MSG.

Big 3

These are the *BIG 3* healthy drugs your body needs! Fish oil, a green supplement, and probiotic supplements are the three supplements that every one must be taking every single day. Make sure your spouse, your children, your parents, and grandparents are taking the *BIG 3* as well. If this is all you change in your lifestyle, it will pay huge dividends throughout your life. You will drastically decrease your chances of developing a lifestyle disease such as cancer, heart disease, diabetes, high cholesterol, chronic fatigue, or fibromyalgia. The *BIG 3* will also help keep your immune system boosted throughout your life thus decreasing common colds, flu's, ear infections and other common, yet preventable maladies.

Healthy Drugs

Fish Oil

Probiotics

Green Drink

Wheat Grass	*Chlorella*	*Broccoli*
Alfalfa	*Spirulina*	*Cauliflower*
Carrot	*Coriander*	*Parsley*
Spinach	*Turmeric*	*Grapeseed*
Blueberries	*Pomegranate*	*Aloe Vera*
Green Tea	*Rosemary*	*Milk Thistle*

Chapter 7

Healthy Eating

Nutrition is another key for your wellness lifestyle that goes hand-in-hand with healthy supplements. Realistically, nutrition is the most important aspect of your health. Whether you want to eat better, you're trying to lose weight, trying to overcome diseases such as diabetes or cancer, or help your child develop a healthier lifestyle; putting the right nutrition into your body is the most important aspect of health and wellness.

There are thousands of diets out right now and hundreds of nutrition books at your local bookstore. Most people are so confused when it comes to a healthy diet, they just don't know where to start. Should you choose a diet that is low carb or high carb? Low protein or high protein? Low fat or high fat diet? They are all out there. You can't help but be confused. Who do you trust? You can't even watch television without seeing a new diet plan or a new supplement on the market that is all the rage and offers the ultimate answer. It's all meant to be very alluring. But what is the right answer?

"If it wasn't here 500 years ago, don't eat it."

The easiest way to remember what to eat and what not to eat is this: *If it wasn't here 500 years ago, don't eat it.* So what does that leave you? It leaves you every single fruit and vegetable on the planet, and anything that grows on this earth. For that matter, it leaves you everything that lives on the earth. So, most of your diet should be from fruits and vegetables, animal meats, fish, nuts, seeds and berries. Simple. Tasty. Super Healthy.

By eating from the earth you will be getting the proper nutrition needs that support the normal biological functions of the body. You will be able to lose weight and better yet, maintain a healthy weight.

Why do so many people that go on a diet lose weight and then balloon back up to an unhealthy weight again? It's because they quit eating foods from the earth. They go back to their favorite restaurants and they start eating processed or packaged foods again.

The human body was not intended to eat anything processed. When you eat processed foods, the preservatives and other chemicals cause problems at the cellular level and your normal cellular functions are disrupted. This is when sickness, disease, and obesity can creep into your life. A healthy diet from the earth will support and maintain the development of healthy bones, muscles, ligaments, tendons and joints. It will also prevent almost every disease that you hear about in America today. Your daily energy level will be tremendously increased. This is what you will probably notice first. The next thing to benefit is your sex drive and your interest to thrive. Do you remember what it felt like to thrive?

None of this is really rocket science. Your body needs the micronutrients, phytonutrients, vitamins, and minerals from the earth to thrive and survive. We have been eating off the earth since the beginning of time. It has only been in recent years, relatively speaking, that farming has become industrialized and foods have become processed with chemicals and preservatives to enhance their shelf life. This is the same reason that in the same era, disease and sickness has skyrocketed.

If our nation would get back to our roots (pun intended), and eat more foods that are farm-to-table, then disease, sickness, hospital and doctor visits, and prescription medicine use would dramatically decrease and there would not be a health care crisis.

> ## "Just because you're not sick, doesn't mean you're healthy."

There is nothing natural about feeding chickens and cattle hormones, steroids and antibiotics. The remnants of the hormones and medicines they give the animals end up on your plate and then in your body. The same goes for farm crops. Pesticides, fungicides and herbicides all end up on your plate, as well. Now scientists are trying to genetically modify our fruits and vegetables, too. Who knows what the health consequences of genetically modified food are going to be? The results probably won't show up for another twenty to thirty years; when it's too late to change the impact it's made on our internal organs.

You can start to make small changes by buying locally grown, organic produce right now and say "no" to GMO (genetically modified foods). Even though it seems cheaper to buy packaged foods now, eventually, you will pay for it with your health. Just because you're not sick, doesn't mean you're healthy.

The price of organic foods is becoming more and more economical. There are alternatives to shopping at an expensive organic grocery store. Dr. Nick has all of his organic fruits and vegetables delivered straight to his doorstep every single week. There are many companies that do this at very reasonable prices. We recommend doing an online search for a company in your area that will do this for you. Having your groceries delivered is a very easy and cost effective way to start serving organic foods to your family.

When Dr. Nick describes the term "eating from the earth", many of his patients tell him that this will be boring and there will not be enough choices. There are plenty of choices. It's not boring, and moreover, there's probably even more variety than you have in your current diet right now. We've included recipes in the back of the book and a quick Internet search will offer you hundreds of more choices for healthy meals.

Super Salads

Adding more salads to your diet is one thing you need to start increasing on a daily basis, and salads alone can be prepared in several different ways. Chopped up vegetables along with nuts or seeds will give you a crunchy, bulky salad that tastes great and really fills you up. Adding on a lean protein such as an organic chicken breast or organic hard-boiled eggs is a great way to add texture and taste to the salad. Adding more vegetables into your menu is really simple. You can add shredded carrots and broccoli to just about every recipe. Replacing cooking liquids with a low sodium vegetable broth adds more nutrition than water, without sacrificing flavor.

Maybe you've heard of Super Foods; we call our *Super Salads* a *Super Meal*. You are getting tons of greens, which is the key to a long life, four-five servings of vegetables, and a lean source of protein. That's all you need!! A recent survey showed 72% of Americans are deficient in their daily vegetable intake, and 83% are deficient in their daily fruit intake. If you could simply change this statistic alone, you would be unbelievably better off. Who knows how this one change alone would affect cancer and heart disease rates?

There are several books that teach you how to sneak more vegetables into your family meals. We're not endorsing hiding the vegetables, instead, you can use these books as a great resource to show you how easy it is to add even more nutrition into your family meals. You don't have to dump all of your favorite family recipes when you find ways to make them more nutritional and less laden with carbohydrates and fats.

Best Meal Of The Day

Many families have a real problem with eating breakfast. They are either *not* eating it, or, they are eating a "sugar breakfast". Examples of a sugar breakfast can be cereal, pancakes, waffles, toast, pastries or sugar-filled coffees and lattes. All of these carbohydrate meals are very bad for your health. Sugars and carbohydrates are the biggest addiction in America and they are the number one cause of our sick and diseased country. Dr. Nick's favorite piece of advice is, "quit putting sugars and carbohydrates into your mouth".

An epidemic is happening in America. Children are fed sugar breakfasts every morning and then they go to school where they struggle to focus on their schoolwork. Then, they are misdiagnosed with Attention Deficit Disorder or Attention Deficit/Hyperactive Disorder. These kids don't have a disease; they are on a sugar high. Their glucose and insulin levels are so out of whack; their little developing brains do not know what is going on. These kids are then put on heavy medication to try to settle them down and they are labeled with a life-long title they can't erase.

Before you take such drastic measures with your own children, clean out all the sugar from their bodies and their meals and watch how positively they respond.

Just like your mother told you, breakfast is the most important meal of the day. Breakfast should consist of protein and antioxidants. Dr. Nick's favorite Super Breakfast is a two-egg veggie omelet. Of course, he chooses organic eggs and organic vegetables that were delivered to his home to make sure he always has healthy ingredients on hand.

To make your own veggie omelet, you can use any veggies you like such as green and red peppers, mushrooms, tomatoes, or broccoli, and make an omelet out of all of it. Dr. Nick washes his omelet down with a *Green Drink* to give his body unlimited energy all throughout the morning and into the afternoon without any caffeine.

Eating From The Earth

Eating from the earth can be very simple and quite fun. You can make a game out of your meal planning and try to get as many Super Foods into each meal and start calling them Super Meals. When grocery shopping, keep to the outside aisles of the grocery store. This is where the fresh fruits and vegetables are. Organic meats and frozen vegetables are also located on the outside of the grocery store aisles.

Stay away from the inside aisles as they only contain packaged and processed foods that contain chemicals, preservatives, and artificial sweeteners. Stay away from artificial sweeteners. They are advertised as low calorie, low carb, or low sugar, but these artificial sweeteners are very dangerous to your body as your body recognizes them as the foreign chemicals that they are. They have been known to have devastating effects on the body and should be avoided at all times.

If you are only eating foods that were here five hundred years ago then you do not have to worry about artificial sweeteners. Otherwise, be on lookout as they are putting these chemicals in virtually every packaged food out there. It's important for your health for you to become an avid label-reader.

Makers of processed foods are counting on you to be ignorant. Education is the most powerful tool you have for bringing more health to your family.

How To Survive Any Party

Don't Go Hungry – Enjoy a *Green Drink*, a protein shake or a healthy meal before heading to the party to keep you from overeating immediately upon arrival.

Limit Alcohol Intake – Alternate every cocktail with a big glass of water to cut down on calorie intake.

3-Bite Rule – Three bites is usually sufficient to satisfy a craving of an unhealthy food.

Portion Control – The size of your palm is a full-serving.

Exercise - Within 12 hours of the party, either before or after.

Chapter 8
Make Time For Dinner

One of the biggest devastations happening to families all across the country is that they are no longer spending time together at the dinner table. Everyone seems too busy to come together for this daily ritual. For many families, dinnertime is the ultimate schedule-buster. You have to plan ahead, prepare the meal long before anyone is hungry, gather the family together for the ten-minute ingestion and clean up the mess afterwards. Who has time for that every single day?

As a mother, Angel understands that it's not completely your fault. In fact, she concedes that children are at the very root of this daily problem. As infants, they started the pattern of eating out on the go. Whenever they cried for hunger, you could easily whip out their bottle or nurse them in an instant. They were immediately satisfied, and in those tender moments of feeding, you were also nourishing their petite souls. You held each other close and bonded. You talked to your baby. You were completely into each other. For a few minutes, you would stop what you were doing. You would find a quiet place, look into your baby's eyes and for a moment in time, you were connected. You were a family.

As they got older, you began to multitask. Your baby could hold their own bottle or somebody else could feed them for you, while you took care of other needs. Fast forward to the days when your children's social calendar has gotten busier than yours. They have school plays, soccer practice, band lessons, karate, you name it, and every single night is packed. You are running Morgan to gymnastics, taking David & John to baseball and in the midst of it all, someone is always starving. "Mom!!! What's for dinner?"

You're already in the car and you are running late because one ballet slipper was missing and the dog ran down the street when you answered your cell phone. What is a mother to do?

According to a 2010 survey, 84% of mothers are choosing to feed their families from a fast-food restaurant at least once every week. Even on the days when everyone is home, the schedule is no less crazy. Helping with homework, running laundry through, catching up on email and bills doesn't leave much time for the family to come together for dinner. So someone brings home take-out and everyone fetches their own, eating while watching TV, studying or standing over the kitchen sink.

Studies have shown that children who eat dinner with their family have less obesity and are overall healthier. Another survey showed there is less drug use in teenagers who consistently eat dinner with their families. Other benefits of eating as a family is that these kids are shown to have better communication skills, superior academic performance, adapt quicker and easier to situations as they mature, and of course, better nutrition and health.

"Behind so many health and social issues in America is the lack of families coming together for dinner."

Every women's magazine is filled with solutions to help with this issue. The latest Stouffer's advertisements tell you that having a real family dinner isn't impossible; you just need a little help.

You didn't get into this bind overnight, and your family won't immediately walk out of their established patterns, but there is hope. Mom, you can make a difference in your children's self-esteem, health, and overall well-being of your entire family when you bring your family back to the dinner table.

Busy mom Stacy says, "With our busy schedules, the only way we can share dinner as a family is if everyone pitches in. The youngest kids set the table, my daughter makes the salad and on Wednesday nights, the guys are in charge. Everyone feels like dinner is something they own." Stacy has taken on the challenge of creating a new legacy for her family.

Very few people have the time or the interest to stand in the kitchen all day long, and you won't have to, either. You can start out with some practical menu plans, institute some help from other family members, and keep the meals simple so that clean up is a snap.

Getting started is half the battle, but it's a battle worth fighting. Family dinner will help fight the battle of the bulge, the battle of sibling rivalry, the battle of communication and the battle of your overall health.

When you plan your meals in advance, you won't be stuck with the high-calorie, high-fat, fast food options in the drive-thru. Even with restaurant menus offering healthier options, you are still consuming a higher amount of sodium, preservatives, calories and fat than you would ever cook up at home. Home cooking is seventy-five percent healthier than restaurant fare, even if you don't cook from scratch. You are in control of the ingredients, and your waistline will thank you for it.

When your family comes together on a daily basis, the sibling bickering is reduced and family communication is greatly improved. Your family will finally have a venue for holding a civil conversation. Mealtime chats can be some of the liveliest and most memorable moments you create for your children.

Turn off the television, iPods and cell phones, and eliminate the outside world while your family comes together, looks each other in the eyes and says "Mom, thanks for cooking!" Even if the words don't come out verbatim, you will see the change in your family's legacy happening right in front of you, at your own dinner table. Don't underestimate the power of your effort. Even if the eye-rolls come out, they are showing you their approval by showing up.

As a bonus, with the money you will save by not eating out, you can take that family vacation this year or add more into your retirement account.

The average family spends about $8.00 per person when they eat out. When you eat at home, the cost is greatly reduced to about $3.00 per person. You can do the math for your own family and see the savings will add up right away. Conservatively, in the first month alone, a family of four can save $400.00. Wouldn't you love to see an extra $400.00 added into your working budget every month? Let alone, the lower costs on prescriptions, doctor's visits, and time missed for being sick.

One change to your day can transform your family legacy. You nourish your family every single day – but if it comes in a wrapper and is hurriedly eaten in the car while everyone is in their own electric-charged world, how much nourishment is really gained?

Chapter 9

Meal Planning

Stopping at the drive-thru for dinner happens when you don't have a plan. Burger joints and taco stops are all banking on you being in a hurry with kids whining in the backseat. We all whine when we are hungry, and having someone else cook and clean up always sounds like a great option, until it becomes a lifestyle problem.

Look at your calendar. For the most part, each week repeats itself. Every Monday is the scout meeting, every Tuesday is this and every Wednesday is that. Most running around is not a surprise. The surprises come when equipment is lost and you're running late and oh, by the way, Jenna just remembered to tell you that you're in charge of bringing snacks tomorrow.

In Angel's home, they schedule time for dinner every night. It goes on the calendar. Meals are planned according to how busy the day is, and every day is busy, busier, or busiest. Rare are the days when there is nothing going on in the Tuccy household.

Busy, Busier, Busiest

Typically, there are only three scenarios you need to plan for; *busy nights* when you are home, *busier nights* when you need a quick meal plan before heading out, and *busiest nights* when you need an emergency meal on the go.

On *busier nights*, Angel's plan is to start cooking and be finished cleaning in thirty minutes. That means, that the meal prep can only be ten to fifteen minutes maximum to allow for fifteen minutes at the table and a few minutes for clean up. Do you remember the crockpot™ you received as a wedding gift?

Pull it out from the back of the cupboard and look up recipes that you can start in the morning and serve at night. Thawing frozen items will speed up your prep time. Fifteen minutes together at the table may not seem significant – but watch as the benefits add up. It's cumulative, kind of like interest rates. The more time you spend together, the more valuable it becomes.

For the *busy nights* when you are home, you can relax on the timing a bit, but you still don't want to overwhelm yourself with lengthy meals. Remember, you are already busy, so keep it simple and think ahead. If you're going to make a casserole, it doesn't take twice the time to make two of them, so make them both at the same time. Cook one tonight, and freeze the other for later. You'll have one less night for clean up and you'll be prepared for the next *busy night*. If you're cooking up ground beef or chicken (organic of course) make a double batch for another night's use. Your family will be amazed at how quickly you can pull a meal together – and you're the hero! All moms could use a few more heroic moments, don't you think?

Making up Chicken Wraps in advance for your *busiest nights* on the go will at least offer you a healthy alternative when you are relegated to eating in the car. You can warm them in the microwave or serve them cold with some veggie sticks and fruit.

The secret to all of this is planning ahead and using up what you already have in stock. Look through your pantry and freezer and see what menu ideas you already have. Make a menu plan for the week and a coordinating grocery list. What nights are you in? What nights are you out? What time will you need to serve dinner? When you make a menu plan, we recommend you only plan for five nights of the week. Reserve one night for going out or entertaining and one night for leftovers to make room in the refrigerator for next week's menu plan. By keeping a night or two in reserve, you ensure that you don't over-plan which can leave you with too many perishable items that end up being wasted.

Make Reservations

Make sure that dinnertime is a part of your daily plan. Reserve the time, just as you would if you made dinner reservations at a restaurant. If you use a calendar to schedule your day, add dinnertime as a reservation to help change your habits.

You don't have to lock yourself into a box that says dinnertime is only at 6:00 p.m. and therefore, it would never work because you have events that start at 6:00 p.m. For your family, maybe dinnertime is right after school, at 4:30 p.m. or later at 8:00 p.m. You have to make it work for your family, and no two families are alike. Ideally, dinner is served around the same time every night, but on some nights, you are going to have to be flexible.

On the nights that you have to be out, choose quick meals that can be prepared simply, and more importantly, cleaned up quickly. The last thing you want to come home to after a long night out is a kitchen full of dirty dishes, so include the clean up time in your plan. When you were growing up, it's very likely that your own mother was the only one who ever cleaned her kitchen, but those days are gone. These days, everyone chips in and the job gets finished with everyone's participation. We don't recommend that you seclude one person to the kitchen duties. It's lonely, sad and will take forever. Include everyone to clear the table, wipe off countertops, load the dishwasher and sweep the floor. Everyone eats and everyone helps.

What Are You Hungry For?

The most common excuse for not planning weekly meals is that you don't know what you'll be hungry for. That's an excuse. The bright side is that your menu plan has flexibility built into it. You can always swap meal plans during the week. Plus, your family will be predictably hungry for tacos when they've been reading about them on the on the menu all week. Put dishes on the menu that you enjoy eating and your excuses will dissolve.

SEXY FOODS

*Green Tea

*Blueberries

*Blackberries

*Strawberries

*Broccoli

*Cauliflower

*Healthy Greens (Kale, Spinach, Romaine)

*Grapefruit

*Tomatoes

*Purple Grapes (Grapes, Grape Juice, Red Wine)

*Red and Green Peppers

*Pumpkin

*Carrots

*Olive Oil

*Whole Grains (Brown Rice, Quinoa, Barley, Oatmeal)

*Almonds & Walnuts

*Fish (Wild Salmon, Black Cod, Sardines)

*Herbs & Spices (Ginger, Cinnamon, Garlic, Onion)

If you look over the Sexy Food list and picture what the foods look like, you will notice it is a very colorful list. You need to be eating a rainbow of colors every day. Make sure to hit almost every color of the rainbow on a daily basis as far as your food choices go. Different colors mean different nutrients. The nutrients of fruits and vegetables are called phytonutrients or phytochemicals. "Phyto" means plant, and of course, we know what nutrient means. In Dr. Nick's office, he refers to phytonutrients as plant nutrients. He tells his patients all the time that they need to be getting an abundance of plant nutrients every single day and better yet, every single meal. If you are not eating enough vegetables throughout the day, then there are phytonutrient supplements on the market. This is what he refers to as a *Green Drink*. This is what Dr. Nick personally eats for lunch every day during the work week. Even if you eat plenty of vegetables throughout the day, a *Green Drink* is great insurance for getting in all the health benefits of phytonutrients each and every day. Fortunately, there are no bad side effects for taking in too many vegetables every day. Your body is very smart. It is designed to keep what it needs and eliminate what it doesn't need on any given day.

You will start to hear more and more about phytonutrients in the coming years as scientists are discovering many different phytonutrients in all types of fruits and vegetables. What you need to know is that you need all different kinds of phytonutrients consistently so don't get hung up on just *one* fruit or *one* vegetable diet. Make sure you are getting all the colors of the rainbow daily - red, orange, yellow, green, blue and purple.

Phytonutrients are super nutrition for your body. They are basically antioxidant, anti-inflammatory, and immune-boosting nutrients that are very powerful and promote many different functions in the body all the way down to the cellular level.

Humans have eaten them since the beginning of time, and they were put on this earth for a reason: for human consumption and to promote health and well-being. Researchers are finally finding out that phytonutrients can help many of the sicknesses and diseases that are running rampant right now.

The Greek philosopher and doctor, Hippocrates (460 BC), who is also known as *The Father Of Medicine,* used leaves, plants and the bark of willow trees to treat fevers and other sicknesses. It is funny now, that health has come full circle, and we are reverting back to these same plant nutrients to treat today's common diseases. Current research shows that at every step along the way to malignancy, plant chemicals tend to reduce the likelihood of transmission to the next stage.

We cannot stress enough how important phytonutrients are. Every single meal needs a variety of color in it. Take the advice of your mother saying, "eat your veggies," and at the very least, try to get a *Green Drink* in every day. Whether it's a workday, a weekend, or even if you are traveling, make an effort to get your *Green Drink*.

Green Drink Recipe

The Juice From Your Vegetable Medley
Or
1 Scoop Green Drink Powder
8 Ounces Of Water

Chapter 10

Reading Your Blood Work

One of the greatest mysteries you will ever face will be to decipher the printout that your doctor gives to you after having your blood work drawn. Being able to read your own blood work is very important. The frequency of having blood work should be done anywhere from every year for healthy individuals to every couple months for people with various sicknesses and diseases. It's important to understand the blood work ranges that are on your lab report are very average. Dr. Nick always tells his patients the ranges the lab reports give you represent a C student. They are very average. We do not want you to be a C student; Dr. Nick wants your blood work to be an A+ student. Below is a chart on how to look at your Lipid panel, which is the most common blood work ordered today. We are not going to get into the cholesterol debate in this book, but just know there are many more important factors that go into heart disease than your cholesterol reading. Dr. Nick is more concerned with his patient's CRP levels (C-Reactive Protein), glucose levels, homocystein levels and Lipoprotein-a levels than cholesterol readings when gauging a patient's heart disease risk. Remember, by taking the *BIG 3* supplements mentioned earlier on a regular basis, eating properly (which means staying away from carbohydrates and sugars), getting the right kind of exercise consistently, and maintaining proper structure and alignment of your body; you should not have any issues with keeping your blood levels in the A+ range.

BLOOD WORK – LIPID PANEL RANGES

Risk Factor	Optimal	Risk	Serious Risk
C-Reactive Protein	<1	>2	>3
Homocysteine	<8	>8	>12
Lipoprotein-A	<10	>11	>25
Fasting Glucose	<100	110-125	>125
Fibrinogen	<235	>235	>350
HDL	>65	<55	<45
Triglycerides (TG)	<100	>100	>150
Fasting Insulin	<2	<5	<10
TG/HDL ratio	1:1	2:1	4:1

BLOOD WORK EXPLANATIONS
AND DEFINITIONS

C-Reactive Protein (CRP) – CRP is an inflammation marker. It is a protein found in the blood that rises when systemic inflammation is raised. Inflammation and CRP are two of the earliest signs we can keep an eye on for future heart disease issues or even a heart attack.

Homocysteine – Elevated homocysteine levels in the blood can cause severe damage to arteries therefore raising your risk for heart attack or stroke. It is a great marker in your blood work to keep an eye on and should never be above 8. Vitamins B6, B12, and folic acid will help clear homocysteine from your blood.

Lipoprotein A (Lipo-A) - Lipo-A is a sticky protein that attaches to bad cholesterol (LDL) and may cause plaques
114

within the arterial walls if levels are too high. This is another great marker for underlying heart disease.

Fasting Glucose – This study shows how quickly and efficiently your body deals with sugar/carbohydrates. If this number is in the risk or serious risk column, you need to take a serious look at what you're eating and drinking on a daily basis. Decreasing consumption of breads, pastas, rice, cereals, and other carbohydrates from your diet will help you optimize your glucose and insulin levels.

Fibrinogen – Elevated fibrinogen means you have thicker blood, which moves less easily through blocked or partially blocked arteries causing an increased risk for heart attacks and strokes.

HDL – Stands for High Density Lipoprotein, otherwise known as your good cholesterol. HDL is a scavenger that grabs loose cholesterol and brings it back to the liver for processing. The more HDL you have the better because this means there are more scavengers out there sweeping up bad cholesterol from your blood stream.

Triglycerides – Triglycerides become elevated in a diet that is high in sugars and carbohydrates. If your triglycerides become elevated, you are at a serious risk for heart disease. Decreasing foods such as bread, pasta, rice and cereals will help keep your triglycerides in optimal range.

Fasting Insulin – Insulin is produced by the pancreas after consuming sugars and carbs and helps eat up the sugar in the bloodstream. Your insulin marker is a way to see how well your pancreas is working. If these numbers are elevated it means too much glucose will be floating around in your blood stream which can cause all these other blood markers to elevate.

116

TG/HDL Ratio – This ratio is one of the most reliable ratios to predict future heart disease issues. A lot of blood work tests do not have this on the printout you receive from your lab or doctor, but it is very easy to do on your own. Ideally, you want a 1:1 ration between your triglycerides and HDL ratio.

Pass On The Salt

Instead of pouring extra salt for flavor, look for ways to include these healthy spices into your meals:

Ginger, Garlic, Chili, Cinnamon, Turmeric, Black Pepper, Oregano, Coriander, Cumin, Mustard, Peppermint

Spices compensate for flavor in your low-fat diet, they have potent antioxidant properties and help slow down the aging process. Spices boost your immune system, fight disease and turn ordinary meals into an extraordinary experience.

Chapter 11

Balanced Exercise Routines

You know that exercise is very good for you. It is absolutely something that you need to be doing every single day. It will help your heart and arteries, keep you looking good in your bathing suit, and fill you with energy. What a lot of people do not know, most likely, are the best specific types of exercise that will give you the most benefits for your health, wellness, and longevity. We will also talk about different types of exercise programs that you should stay away from because they might actually do more harm than good. In fact, most people are actually exercising the wrong way. When Dr. Nick goes to the gym, he typically sees people causing their bodies more harm even though they think they are doing something good for themselves. Worse than not exercising is doing the wrong exercise.

What is the most balanced and effective way the human being is supposed to exercise? Just like our food motto is, *if it wasn't here 500 years ago, don't eat it*, the same is sort of true with exercise. To find out the most beneficial types of exercises that you can do to promote health and longevity, you must look at your ancestors. Most of them were hunters and gatherers. This type of lifestyle demanded a lot of physical exertion and movement. Their daily exercise consisted of walking and running in search of food. They would walk for a while, climb, swim, and sprint after wild animals, such as buffaloes. If you asked yourself what type of exercise we just explained, it can be classified as cross-training exercise. Studies of these ancestral hunters and gathers show very little to no signs of cardiovascular disease, which is one of the top killers in America today. This can be attributed not only to their daily types of exercise, but also to their diet, which was free of

120

sugars, carbohydrates, and processed foods. Creating a healthy lifestyle is not complicated, even with our updated American conveniences.

As a human population, we have evolved immensely from the hunting and gathering days, but since genetics takes so many years to evolve, we should still be exercising just like we did many years ago. Back then, their very livelihood could depend on being able to sprint away from a predator or sprint toward an animal for the kill. If you don't get the kill, you simply do not eat that day. It was a very high-intensity type of training back then. Of course, you do not have to worry about sprinting for your life anymore, but your exercise regime should still reflect the lives of your ancestors. It should consist of high-intensity sprint workouts and resistance exercises. You should also be looking for new challenges and new types of exercise in order to keep your body challenged. If we were truly hunters and gatherers, we would not be doing the exact same movements and physical exercises day in and day out. So what makes you think that using the same machines at your local health club every Monday, Wednesday, and Friday would be beneficial? You definitely need to keep mixing things up, but overall, you need to focus on sprint or interval exercises coupled with resistance training.

The human body is not meant to run or exercise for long distances. The prestigious medical journal, *Circulation*, did a study on Boston marathon runners. The study tested sixty runners in the 2004 and 2005 Boston marathons. They did pre and post heart studies, such as echocardiographs, on the runners. The study concluded that completion of a marathon is associated with correlative biochemical and echocardiograph evidence of cardiac dysfunction and injury, and this risk is *increased* in those participants with less training. Simply put, running twenty-six miles causes *irreversible damage* to your heart. Remember, the human body is not designed for this. By
122

no means are we advocating *not* exercising, but we do want to stress the proper types of exercise that will benefit you the most for your own health, wellness, and longevity.

A great example of this point is Jim Fixx, an American icon among marathon runners. He was the author of the best-selling 1977 book, *The Complete Book of Running*. He moved millions of Americans to get off their butts and start exercising. Of course, he was pushing Americans to run and jog long distances. We commend him for his efforts to get us off our butts and moving. This was a very good thing for America. However, Fixx, an avid long-distance runner, died of a heart attack at the age of fifty-two years *young*. Due to the fact that he was performing exercise that was actually detrimental to his health and his immune system, Fixx only lived half of his life.

Besides taking a toll on your heart, long-distance training also places a huge burden on your joints—specifically your ankles, knees, and hip joints. In Dr. Nick's practice, he has come across many long-distance runners that have severe arthritis in these joints and even total joint replacements at the young ages of forty, fifty, and sixty years old. The daily wear and tear on these joints from hitting the pavement for long distances over the years takes a major toll on the cartilage within the joints. The cartilage in your joints acts as a shock absorber between your bones. Every step you take wears down those shock absorbers a little more and a little more. So if you are running long distances, especially on the pavement for many years, you will wear down those shock absorbers much more quickly and speed up the arthritis process. That is why we see many middle-aged patients, with worn-down joints such as hips and knees. Sometimes, the only option is to get an artificial joint.

The moral of the story is that the body is supposed to be able to handle physical exertion and physical exercise. When you perform an activity over and over again that the body is not supposed to be doing in the first place, it is going to cause problems. Maybe not right away, but eventually you will experience side effects. If you do more specific interval-type training, the joints of your body will be able to hold up and perform pain free at age 100. Do the activities that you are designed to do and you will be better off for it.

Sprinting vs. Running

Now that we have gone over how our ancestors got their "exercise" many years ago, let's dig in and really discover what you should be doing today. We really don't imagine you sprinting after buffalo and killing them with your swords or spears, but we're certain you've watched the Olympic Games at some point in your life. We're going to compare a one-hundred-yard sprinter to a long-distance runner, as seen in the games. The sprinters are always very lean, muscular, and look very healthy. You can see every muscle fiber in their bodies, as they have no body fat, basically everything you want to look like when bikini season rolls around. The long-distance runners look skinny as well, but they look like an unhealthy skinny. They usually look frail, their eyes are sunken in, they look malnourished, and do not look like the healthiest people overall. The difference between these two types of athletes is that one is exercising just like the human body is designed to exercise and the other is actually causing harm to his or her body with an exercise regime.

Let's dig a little deeper into these two different kinds of training. The long-distance trainer wakes up every morning, puts on running shoes, and hits the open road. The runner might spend an hour or more for a morning run and then do it all over again at night. This is both unhealthy and detrimental to your body. First of all, every time you exercise, you are creating free radicals in your body. Free radicals are not good and actually cause things like cancer and heart disease. Now, the overall benefits from exercise are still good, but every type of exercise does and will cause the production of free radicals inside our bodies. That is why there are different types of exercise that are good and other types of exercise that actually do more harm than good. When you are performing long-distance exercise and putting in mile after mile, your body produces an enormous amount of free radicals. It is almost as if the body goes into survival mode when you have an exercise regime like this. Year after year and mile after mile, you are putting a lot more pressure on your body. Dr. Nick has treated many baby boomers who have been running long distances for years. Many have run year after year for forty to fifty years. All of these patients are now coming in with knee, hip, ankle, and low back pain caused by the pressure of running for all those years. Can you imagine the pounding these joints have taken over the decades? He cannot even help many of these patients and has to refer them out for knee and hip replacements. Trust us, if you can help it, you want to keep your own knee and hip joints, versus replacing them with an artificial stainless steel joint. These human-made artificial joints will never be as good as the ones your parents gave you.

We are not saying that these patients made a huge mistake by wanting to run and exercise all their lives. We commend them for doing so, but they need to stop their way of training right now and get to a more interval-based training. Nobody knew years ago that there were more beneficial types of training out there. A few decades ago, running long distance was the thing to do, and we thought it was the fountain of youth. Now, however, research has caught up, and we realize there is a better way. Remember, at one point in time, we also didn't know that cigarettes were bad for us. Overall, it is okay that the "jogging fad" hit America. It at least made us start thinking about exercise. Now, we need to take it a step further, and really get specific about exercise and start a program that will best serve our bodies.

This takes us to interval training, or sprint training. This is how our Olympic sprinters have been training for years, and it is exactly how the hunters and gatherers lived their daily lives many years ago. You are not going to need an expensive trainer or a high-tech stopwatch to start your interval training program. As a matter of fact, you will not need any equipment that you do not have right now. All you really need is a mind-set that you are going to switch up how you perform your daily exercises. Most treadmills, bikes, and elliptical machines already have an interval regime programmed into them. Interval routines are set up to go really hard for one minute, then relax for a couple minutes, and keep repeating that sequence for twenty to twenty-five minutes. This type of training is actually going to save a lot of distance runners many hours per week, and you'll definitely see the results both physically and mentally. Your heart, lungs, and joints are also going to reap the benefits.

Dr. Nick's Personal Training Regimen

An example of interval training that I personally do is going to our neighborhood park and doing 10 sets of 15-second hill sprints. There is a nice hill that takes me about 15 seconds to sprint up. I then turn around and slowly walk to the bottom of the hill which takes me about one minute. By the time I reach the bottom I have completely caught my breath. I then turn back up the hill and sprint to the top as fast as I possibly can. I usually do this about 10-15 reps, which takes about 25 minutes.

Every time I walk into my local health club, I cringe when I see the whole line of treadmills with people either walking or jogging at a low-intensity pace. I just want to kick them in high gear and into interval training.

Stay away from the long three to four-mile jogs outside and the easy thirty to forty-five minute jaunts on the elliptical machine;

start moving toward shorter workouts with higher intensity, and your body is going to respond like it never has before.

Muscle Training

Along with the interval-type cardio training, the second aspect of this type of training is resistance training. You need to be working your muscles. All the muscles of your body need to be challenged. Every time a muscle is worked, it burns up sugar. This means less glucose floating around in our bloodstream wreaking havoc on your body's daily processes. Training your muscles keeps your overall bone structure healthier and reduces the impact of osteoporosis.

Muscle training can be done at the gym using weights and resistance bands or be done at home using your own body weight against yourself. Push-ups, pull-ups, stair climbing, and crunches are all designed to use your own body weight against itself, providing muscle training.

You can cut the amount of time spent at the gym in half, and see twice the results. Not only will you see the results within your body, but your body will also reap the longevity benefits that you aren't seeing.

With the combination of interval training and resistance training, you will burn more calories, lose more fat, start to see lean muscle tissue that is hidden right now, and improve cardiovascular health tremendously.

It probably sounds almost too good to be true. You can see all of these results, while spending less time at the gym. It is that easy. There is a reason why millions of people are spending so much time at the gym and not getting tremendous health benefits out of it. Instead of thinking of going to the gym as "social time" use the time more constructively. Trust us, you are going to be working much harder than you have been. Your heart rate will be higher and you will be breathing much more rapidly than your normal routine. The difference is that you will decrease the amount of time you spend at the gym.

Below is a sample of interval "hill sprints" that you can use. Plugging in a treadmill, bike, or stair stepper are definitely other great exercises, but we want you to get the idea of the time frame and intensity. The workout is started and finished with a three- to five-minute slight jog and stretching.

Interval Training Schedule

Week	Reps	Work	Recovery	Total Workout Time
1	6	60-sec. hill sprint	walk (2 mins)	18 minutes
2	8	60-sec. hill sprint	walk (2 mins)	24 minutes
3	10	60-sec hill sprint	walk (1.5 mins)	25 minutes
4	10	45-sec. hill sprint	walk (1.5 min)	22.5 minutes

This chart shows the general idea of how you can start doing interval training. Total workout time goes from eighteen minutes to twenty-two and a half minutes, but rather than just going out for a nice little jog for twenty-five minutes, you are going really hard with enough rest to recover. On a lot of the treadmills and other cardio machines now, you can actually program this type of work out into the menu. This makes it really easy to jump on the machine and start your interval routine at the gym. If you're an outside runner or biker, find a location where you'll be doing your intervals and you are ready to go. For the really cold days when you don't want to climb out of bed, making love is a great interval workout.

Chapter 12

No More Excuses

Gaining one pound is not a big deal. Over the course of time, one pound is hardly noticeable. One pound every year, however, and your jeans don't fit any more. So, you buy one size up. A few babies or years later, and it's only natural to have to buy the next size larger. Then one day, you notice your rear end in a three-way mirror and it's not pretty. Thank goodness for the fashion trend of longer sweaters. Maybe no one will notice. If you pair an oversized shirt with some leggings, you can be sneaky about your fat. Ten years pass, fifteen, even twenty and there is just no reason to ever think you can be pre-baby weight ever again.

All those fabulous looking Hollywood stars with their flat abs and toned thighs only look that way because they hire personal trainers and bring in private chefs. You know that you could look like that too, if only you had someone to motivate you to exercise and then take care of all your dietary needs. If only.

You already know that the experts suggest thirty minutes of exercise every day. It's good for your heart. It's good for eliminating toxins out of the body and warding off life-killing diseases. It gives you more energy, improves your skin tone and keeps your muscles firm and your waistline trimmed. Exercising sets a great example for your children. There are probably a million reasons to exercise. And yet, you still don't do it.

Why you should exercise is not even a question people ask anymore. You already know why, but a lot of people do not know which types of exercises are the most beneficial, and which exercises will bring you the quickest results. Maybe you've cried along with the big losers on the television series, and you've probably consoled a girlfriend or two about her weight struggles. I'm sure you've tried all the diet fads and yet you are still struggling with your weight. Even if you aren't concerned with the number on the scale, maybe you get winded carrying groceries in from the car or have trouble bringing a load of laundry up the stairs.

Lack of exercise is taking its toll on your body at a rate that you can't control anymore. When you were young, you could eat anything you wanted and not gain an inch. When you were young, you were probably far more active than you are now. You danced, you played in the park, you hiked, you rode bikes, and you walked everywhere when you didn't have a car. In your early years of marriage, you were having sex far more often. You were actively chasing around a toddler. Now, you need to be intentional about incorporating physical activity into your day, and that feels like work. It's not nearly the same as going out dancing until two in the morning, but who wants to pay a babysitter every weekend while you go out and rumba?

There is a perfect exercise designed just for you. You need a simple workout that includes muscle strengthening and cardio and that fits into your busy lifestyle. Ideally, you need something that brings you immediate results.

It's easy to add more physical activity into your day when you enjoy it. What do you love to do that doesn't feel like work but actually puts a smile on your face? Is it yoga, dancing, hiking, swimming, or walking in fundraising races? Yes, lunges are great for working on your thighs, but if they make you frown, take up kickboxing instead. Make sure that whatever you choose to do makes you happy to do it. You are so much prettier when you are smiling than when you are frowning. You are also so much prettier when you try on a pair of jeans in the next size smaller than what you are currently wearing. That is the best smile of all! Hard work pays off. When it comes to exercising, your muscles have memory, so if you had any muscle tone in your previous life, it will come back quickly.

"Eat Better. Exercise Better."

The easiest strategy for losing weight is to eat better and exercise better. Easier said than done, but start by saying it. Give yourself a goal, make a plan and write it down.

"I am eating healthier."

"I am losing those extra ten pounds."

"I am setting a healthy example for my family."

You don't have to run out to the local gym and sign up for an annual membership. Start by taking a brisk walk after lunch and dinner. Ten minutes of intense walking that raises your heart rate will feel great. Take someone with you and ten minutes will easily turn into twenty. Plus, you'll have a great conversation. A quick interval training session in the morning before your shower only takes twenty-five minutes and works out every muscle group in your body. Watch your arms become more defined and gorgeous. Notice how your thighs feel stronger and fit in your pants so much nicer. Smile and say thank you when your gal pals tell you look great.

Change Your Answer

When your girlfriends call and say let's go to the mall, suggest going to a dance class instead. Everyone will have a great time and your budget will thank you. Just being at the mall encourages you to spend money on items you didn't even know you needed, and then you have to come home and find a new home for all of your purchases. Your shopping hobby turns into a disorganized mess at home.

Get Organized

Studies have proven that you spend sixty minutes a day looking for lost items. When you reduce how much stuff comes into your home and it will be much easier to get organized. When you are more organized, you will find the extra time in your day that you can use to exercise. What would you do with an extra hour every day? You could completely change your physique. You will feel more attractive. When you feel more attractive, your loved ones will notice. Think about how that will improve your sex life!

Have Fun

Sign up for local events – charity bike rides, 5K runs, walks and stair climbs all offer great ways to get involved in your community and hang out with friends. This also gives you the extra boost of motivation to get out and train for the events. You'll push yourself to stay accountable. You don't want to be the one that falls behind. Inside everyone is a little competitive streak to do well, so you'll be motivated to be prepared so you can keep up with your friends. You can do a web search for the local events and then ask your friends to join you. Set up times to do interval training together. Before you know it, exercise is part of your regular routine.

Once you find small ways to bring more activity into your day, you might be surprised at how easy it is to find more.

Turn up the music and dance with your kids. Sure, at first, they might think you're crazy, but they will join you. When they pull out the Wii, play along with them. Rather than sit on the bench when you take them to the park, bring along a ball to play with them. Don't sit in your car and wait for them to come out of their class, park far away and walk to meet them. Just for kicks, leave the car at home and walk or ride your bikes to some of your weekend errands. Avoid the front parking spots and park in the last spot. Take the stairs instead of the elevator. Turn off the television and go for a walk. Practice yoga in the morning and before bed. Make it a game. Make it a race. Make it active and you'll make it fun.

Celebrate Success

Reward yourself for your good behavior. For every minute that you are active, put a dime or a quarter in a reward jar. Save up for a great outfit, or a date or whatever motivates you. It's up to you to stop making excuses. If you find yourself saying "I don't have time" put a dollar in an excuse jar. Donate the money to a charity. This is not a reward for you. Isn't it time you took charge of your own life and stopped making excuses? You wouldn't accept those lame excuses from anyone else. Be in charge of your life. Eat right and exercise right.

Put It On The Calendar

Write your exercise plans in your calendar as if it were an appointment. Schedule it and protect it. It's really easy to keep this date with yourself when you tell others, "I'm sorry, I already have an appointment at that time." Once you commit to it, it won't fall on the back burner, but as long as you keep offering yourself a way out, you will never fit it in. It's up to you to change your family legacy.

Be Intentional

They say it takes forty-five days to change a habit, and you're on the ninety-day plan to create a new lifestyle. In order to stop an old behavior, you have to replace it with something new. If you have a bad habit you are working to change, rather than planning to stop cold-turkey, find a new and improved habit to replace it with.

144

Based on the five stages of change, you've already entered into the *Effort Stage.*

"There is a happy person buried underneath

all your stress. "

When you start to add more activity into your routine, make a plan for the entire next week. What activities will you do? When will you do them? Make sure you have all the equipment and resources, and then put it in your calendar. You could lose ten-twenty inches in twenty days, depending on your activity level. Doesn't that excite you? Isn't it motivating to know that by the end of the month, you could be back in those jeans that you have stashed in the back of the closet? Aren't you excited to know that you will be able to keep up with your kids on the playground and be the envy of all the housewives sitting on the benches? You will glow. You will smile more. You will be

145

happier with your physique. There is a happy person buried underneath all of that stress – go get her!

WEEKLY EXERCISE SCHEDULE

SUN | MON | TUES | WED | THURS | FRI | SAT

Often times, because your body is changing slowly every day, you won't even notice the improvements. So, before you change your intention, weigh yourself and take your body measurements. Measure your chest, arms, waist, hips, and thighs. Keep track and you'll be pleasantly surprised at the results. When you start out, set a seven-day goal. Then set another seven-day goal. Take it one step at a time until you've created a new lifestyle for yourself.

MEASUREMENTS

DAY 1 | DAY 7 | DAY 14 | DAY 21 | DAY 28

Give yourself the gift of exercise. It is the true gift that keeps on giving. Ten, twenty, thirty days from now, you can snub your trim thighs at all of the Hollywood stars – you've come a long way, baby!

No More Excuses

Change Your Answer

Get Organized

Have Fun

Celebrate Success

Put It On The Calendar

Be Intentional

Exercise Everyday

Track Your Improvement

Chapter 13

A Balanced Structure

Hippocrates (The Father Of Medicine) once stated that we should look at the human body frame first when looking for a cure to common maladies. He stated this over 2,000 years ago, and it still stands true today. Without a proper frame and a proper structure you will never be as healthy as you want to be. This is where regular chiropractic care, massage therapy, yoga, pilates and other bio-mechanical modalities come into play to get your body working optimally.

Chiropractic is the most misunderstood health profession in the world. Chiropractors are still looked at as back and neck pain doctors, which is very unfortunate. This is far from the truth, and it is unfortunate that people still don't understand that we are nervous system doctors. Chiropractic is the science, art, and philosophy of removing nerve pressure from the body.

Nerve pressure happens to everyone and it is caused by life's daily stresses. Those stresses can be physical, emotional and chemical. Physical stress can be anything from lifting heavy boxes, picking up your kids and taking them in and out of car seats. Even sitting at a computer all hunched over is a physical stress.

"Prepare your body for the stresses that life throws at you."

Chemical stresses are all the toxins you put into your body through your foods and drinks, and emotional stresses are those things you worry about on a day-to-day basis. These three different types of stresses slowly weaken you each day by putting pressure on your nervous system. Think of nerve pressure as stress on the spinal column.

No matter how old you are, how active or inactive you are, or what your occupation is, you have stress on your nervous system. There is no way you can avoid stress and Dr. Nick never tells his patients that he is going to reduce their stresses. He wants to make your body and your structure strong enough so you can deal with the stresses life throws at you. Your body is a lot like your car: the better you treat it, the longer it is going to last. Going to your chiropractor on a regular basis and getting a wellness adjustment is just like giving your car an oil change and having a maintenance check-up. Unfortunately, many people take better care of their cars than they take care of their own body. Chiropractic care is a habit you need to take part in on a regular basis to help keep your body de-stressed and the structure of your spine and nervous system maintained.

The nervous system is a very vital component to your health

and longevity. It is the control center of your entire being. The nervous system is made up of your brain, spinal cord, and all the hundreds of nerves that run throughout your body and control every cell, tissue, organ and function of your body. Picture it as a circuit board with all the connections and wires intertwined. If one connection is broken, the information cannot get from point A to point B and the circuit cannot carry out is function.

This is essentially how the body works. The brain constantly sends signals down the spinal cord and out through an intertwined network of nerves until it reaches its destination point and controls some type of function in the body. For example, if you want to move your fingers to type an email, your brain will send a signal to your neck; your neck will then send a signal down a nerve to your hand and fingers and you will be able to move your fingers and type an email. This is your nervous system at work. More importantly, every second

152

of your life, your brain will send a signal down your spinal cord to your heart and tell your heart to beat. This happens whether you are awake, sleeping, working, or watching TV. Your nervous system never sleeps, and this control center of your body is the most important system inside you. It is your chiropractor's job to keep it running efficiently if you want to live a long and healthy life. It all starts with keeping your spine aligned.

If there is any static or pressure anywhere within your spine or musculoskeletal system, your nervous system slows down and will become compromised. You might feel this as joint pain or inflexibility, but it is much more than that. This is why regular chiropractic care is so important. Chiropractic care will maintain the integrity of your structural system and keep your nerves working optimally. This is just as important, if not more important than eating properly and exercising the right way. Your spine is what keeps your body rockin' and rollin'.

Dr. Nick has had many patients tell him that as they started their chiropractic care, they noticed they did not get the colds, flu's, or sinus infections that they have so long been prone to. Most of these people came to his office originally for neck and back pain, but as they started working with their nervous system, their entire health and immune system was extremely boosted. It always puts a smile on Dr. Nick's face when these patients relay to him the great side effects of chiropractic care. You will feel better on the outside, and everything on the inside will function better too!

Chiropractic is leading the wellness revolution that is taking place in America. The nervous system is the most important system of the body, and should be the first system taken care of when starting to take back control of your health. Many other professions are now teaching and preaching this "mind-body connection" or "brain-body connection," and it is so great to see America finally wake up and see this is probably the most

154

see America finally wake up and see that this is probably the most important part of being healthy for a long time. Make sure you find a chiropractor that understands the importance of the nervous system, the mind-body connection, and is not just concerned with your temporary back pain.

*Keep Your Family Healthy**

Plan Menus

Shop And Cook Together

Eat Together As Often As Possible

Provide Cut Up Fruits And Vegetables For Easy Snacking

Consume Healthy Supplements

Limit Television Time

Find Games or Classes That Get You Moving Together

Take Family Walks Or Bike Rides

Eliminate Your Own "Fat" Talk.

Speak Positively About Your Own Body

Speak Positively About Each Other's Bodies

*LetsMove.gov

Chapter 14

Super Recipes

By keeping the menu plan on a magnetic pad on the front of the refrigerator door, everyone in the family is in on the secret. They all know where to look for their insatiable need of the daily question: "What's for dinner?" They can even help start a pot of rice, take items out of the freezer to thaw, and if nothing else, it keeps them from hassling you about it. Having the menu posted is comforting for the entire family. You aren't taken by surprise. You don't have to struggle to be creative with your meal ideas while everyone around you is pressuring you to serve them right away. You have a plan. Everyone is in on the plan. Life, at least in this area, is calm. You can breathe and know that you are nourishing your family in more ways than one. Way to go, Mom!

Post your Super Menu on the front of your fridge every week. Use it to make your grocery shopping list. Here is a sample Super Menu:

SUPER MENU

Monday – *Busy Night* – Oriental Chicken With Vegetables

Tuesday – *Busier Night* - Chili In The CrockPot™

Wednesday – *Busiest Night* – Chicken Wraps

Thursday – *Busy Night* - Leftovers

Friday – *Busier Night* – Naked Burgers With Fridge Salad

Saturday – *Busy Night* – Easy Tacos

Sunday – Family Brunch – Casserole from the freezer

Quick and Easy Recipes For Busier Nights

These recipes were chosen for their minimal ingredients and easy kitchen clean up.

Oriental Chicken and Vegetables with Rice

4 oz chicken breast, sliced, per person
2 cups of cooked brown rice (cooked in vegetable broth)
2 cups vegetables – choose 3 different colors
½ cup onion
3 tbsp ginger
3 tbsp soy sauce

Stir-fry chicken, then add vegetables and ginger. Cook until tender. Add soy sauce. Serve over brown rice.

Chicken Chili in Crockpot™

1 can chili beans
1 can black beans
1 can pinto beans
1 cooked chicken breast, chopped
½ cup chopped green bell pepper
½ cup chopped onion
8 ounces tomato sauce
3 tbsp chili seasoning mix
Cover with water or vegetable broth

Add all ingredients to crockpot™ for 8 hours on low, or 4 hours on high.

Chicken Wraps with Rice and Beans

4 oz chicken breast, broiled, per person
2 tbsp salsa per tortilla
1 low-fat whole wheat tortilla per person
1 can black beans
1 tsp chili powder
2 cups of cooked brown rice (cooked in vegetable broth)

Toss rice, chili and beans together. Arrange with the chicken and salsa on tortilla. This can be made with or without chicken. You can make them in advance and keep in the fridge. Warm in the microwave or eat cold for a healthy emergency dinner on the run. You can wrap them in foil and freeze them. Thaw the night before and heat in the oven for 30-minutes (350 degrees) to bring along to a picnic.

Naked Burgers

1 ¼ pound ground beef
½ cup chopped onion
½ cup chopped bell peppers
1 egg
garlic, oregano and pepper, to taste
1 cup tomato salsa
lettuce leaves

Mix ground beef with onion and peppers, spices and egg. Grill patties and top with tomato salsa and lettuce leaves.

Side Salad

For each salad, place a handful of spinach, a scoop of tomatoes and sprinkle with almonds. Lightly drizzle with dressing.

Easy Tacos

1 ¼ pound ground beef, turkey or chicken
½ cup chopped onion
3 tbsp taco seasoning
2 cups of cooked rice – cooked in vegetable broth
Chopped tomato
Chopped spinach
Taco shells, soft or hard

Cook ground meat with onion. Stir in seasoning and cooked rice. Serve in taco shells garnished with tomato and spinach.

Super Fridge Salad

This is perfect for the end of the week, using up all those extra perishables you have left in the fridge.

Top 1 cup of lettuce greens with whatever you have (tomatoes, apples, hard-boiled eggs, nuts, grapes, citrus fruit, berries, leftover fish or chicken, carrots, broccoli, peppers, beans and mushrooms.

Ultra Broth (from the Ultimate Simple Diet)

For an easy way to add more nutrition to your menu, you can keep a jar of Ultra Broth in the fridge to replace the water or liquid in recipes. You can also warm it up and drink as an anytime nutritious energy boost. A box of low-sodium organic vegetable broth also works well. This is a great detoxifying drink when you're "cleansing".

Makes approximately 8 cups or 2 quarts.

3 quarts of water
1 large chopped onion
2 sliced carrots
1 cup white radish root and tops
1 cup winter squash cut into large cubes
1 cup of root vegetables: turnips, parsnips, and rutabagas for sweetness
2 cups of chopped greens: kale, parsley, beet greens, collard greens, chard, dandelion, or cilantro
2 celery stalks
½ cup of seaweed: nori, dulse, wakame, kelp, or kombu
½ cup of cabbage
4 - ½ inch slices of fresh ginger
2 cloves of whole garlic, not chopped or crushed
Sea salt to taste
1 cup fresh or dried shitake mushrooms if available for their powerful immune-boosting properties.

Add all ingredients and place on a low boil for 60 minutes. It may take a little longer. Simply continue to boil to taste. Cool and strain. Throw out the cooked vegetables and keep the broth. Store the broth in a large, tightly sealed glass container in the fridge. Heat gently and drink at least 3-4 cups a day for one week.

The broth is a filling snack that will provide your body with healing nutrients and make it easy for you to detoxify, lose weight and feel great. Consume the broth for 7 days then discard.

Super Breakfast Meals

Broccoli Omelet

2 whole eggs
½ cup of broccoli

Scrambled Eggs With Turkey & Tomato

2 whole eggs
½ cup chopped tomato
3 thin slices of deli turkey breast meat

Tomato & Mushroom Omelet

2 whole eggs
½ cup chopped tomatoes
½ cup sliced mushrooms

Cottage Cheese With Berries

1 cup cottage cheese
½ cup raspberries
½ cup blueberries

Broccoli Omelet with Feta Cheese

2 whole eggs
½ cup of broccoli
1/2 cup shredded feta cheese

Yogurt Breakfast

1 cup non-fat yogurt
top with ¼ cup granola
½ cup blueberries

Mango Protein Smoothie

1 cup milk
1 cup frozen mango chunks
1 scoop protein powder

2-Egg Veggie Omelet

2 whole eggs
1 cup of your favorite chopped vegetables

Berry Protein Smoothie

1 cup milk
1 cup frozen berries
1 scoop protein powder

Green Drink Recipe

The Juice From Your Vegetable Medley
OR 1 Scoop Green Drink Powder
8 Ounces Of Water

Super Lunch Meals

Turkey & Avocado Wrap

3 slices of deli turkey
1 whole wheat tortilla
2 slices tomato
1 oz avocado
dash of black pepper
2 leaves of romaine or spinach lettuce

Turkey & Hummus Pita

3 slices lean turkey
1 small low-fat whole wheat pita
1 tbls hummus
2 slices tomato
4 lettuce leaves
1 tsp mustard

Salmon Salad

4 oz salmon
¼ cup red onion
½ cup chopped bell pepper
½ cup shredded carrots
1 cup spinach
drizzle with olive oil & vinaigrette dressing

Blackened Chicken Breast Salad

1 whole chicken breast
½ cup cucumbers
½ cup tomatoes
¼ cup chopped red onion
1 cup romaine lettuce
1 tbls Italian dressing

Chunky Vegetable Soup

1 cup vegetable broth
½ cup chopped onion
½ cup chopped cabbage
½ cup chopped carrots
½ cup sliced mushrooms

Peanut Butter Banana Protein Smoothie

1 cup milk
1 tbls peanut butter
½ banana
1 scoop protein powder

Super Salad

1 cup lettuce greens
4 oz lean protein (salmon, chicken, turkey, hard-boiled eggs)
1 ½ cups sliced and chopped vegetables (3 varieties)
sprinkle with nuts or berries
lightly drizzle with oil & vinegar

Tuna Salad

5 oz tuna
1 cup shredded romaine or spinach
½ chopped onion
2 tsp mustard
1 tbls olive oil
1 chopped tomato

Black Bean & Mango Salad

1 can black beans
1 chopped mango
2 chopped kiwis
1 cup romaine lettuce
½ cup cilantro
drizzle with lime juice & olive oil

Organic Chili

1 lb ground organic turkey
½ cup celery
½ cup onion
½ cup bell pepper
Can of black beans
Can of chili beans
1 cup diced tomatoes
1 can tomato paste
3 tbls chili seasoning

Turkey Burgers with Grilled Vegetables

3 oz cooked ground turkey
2 slices tomato
1 slice onion
2 leaves romaine lettuce
mustard & ketchup to taste

Chicken Kebabs with Brown Rice

3 oz chicken breast
1 chunked red onion
1 chunked yellow bell pepper
cherry tomatoes
mushrooms
drizzle with olive oil, garlic & pepper

Grilled Ahi Tuna Salad

4 oz tuna steak
2 cups arugula
½ cup sesame seeds
black pepper
sliced pineapple
top with lime vinaigrette

Baked Red Snapper with Broccoli

3 oz baked red snapper with olive oil, garlic & pepper
1 cup steamed broccoli

Serve with side salad
2 cups shredded lettuce drizzled with olive oil & vinegar

Grilled Chicken Breast & Salad

3 oz chicken breast
1 cup lettuce
2 cups of your favorite chopped vegetables (carrots, celery, cucumbers, avocado, bell peppers, tomatoes, etc.)

Grilled Steak with Sweet Baked Potato

3 oz grilled steak with olive oil, garlic & pepper
1 steamed sweet potato
Top with cinnamon and olive oil

Chapter 15

Checklists

Weekly Menu Plan
Plan your menu every week and post it on your fridge.

Sunday |

Monday |

Tuesday |

Wednesday |

Thursday |

Friday |

Saturday |

Weekly Shopping List

Look through your pantry and plan menus from your inventory. Reserve dinnertime on your calendar.

Weekly Exercise Plan

Develop a "week at a glance" exercise plan that includes a variety of activities. Include interval workouts mixed with resistance workouts at least 5 days each week. Refer back to Chapter 11 for an interval training routine.

Sunday |

Monday |

Tuesday |

Wednesday |

Thursday |

Friday |

Saturday |

MEASUREMENTS

DAY 1 | DAY 7 | DAY 14 | DAY 21 | DAY 28

CHEST

ARMS

WAIST

HIPS

THIGHS

WEIGHT

Chapter 16

Plan for Success

In the book *Your Plan For A Balanced Life,* Dr. Rippe recommends six paths for success: kick the procrastination habit, set realistic goals, tap into your personal power, think positively, plan ahead and live in the present.

Kick The Procrastination Habit

Take one small step today rather than tomorrow. A good plan today is far better than having a perfect plan tomorrow. Move from the *Thinking Stage* to the *Effort Stage*.

Set Realistic Goals

Consider your current activity level before jumping into a big exercise regiment. Start with adding a little more activity every single day. Losing one pound a week is very realistic. Schedule interval training and reserve time for dinner.

Tap Into Your Personal Power

The only thing holding you back is you. It's not your schedule. It's not your responsibilities. Your excuses are all in your head. Believe in what you are capable of achieving. Your body is designed to be healthy, despite genetics. Your lifestyle determines your health factor.

Think Positively

Your new lifestyle will have peaks and valleys and some times will be easier than others. Cycling through the stages is a natural part of your progress. Forge through the tough times and give yourself credit for the positive changes you've made in the good times. You can do this. You have all the resources you need to make the healthy changes a possibility. Look at the big picture and recognize that your family will be better off in the future and your future starts right now.

Plan Ahead

If you plan for success, you cannot fail. Set a goal for yourself and write the baby steps down. If you don't write it down, it will be easier for you to put off and skip out on the positive changes that are waiting for you. Success is waiting for you in your future and even though you can't live in the past, sometimes progress is easier viewed in the rearview mirror. On occasion, look back to see how far you've come.

Live In The Present

The goal of planning ahead is to allow you to free up the present moment versus worrying about what happened in the past or what's coming down the pike. You can't change the past. You've planned for the future, so you can stop worrying about it. Live in the present. Live your healthiest life.

Reaching your potential is the ultimate goal. You have a chance to make a difference in other people's lives. If everyone does a little something, you'll discover big changes are waiting for you.

Chapter 17

Resources

Premier Chiropractic & Natural Medicine, P.C.
Dr. Nick Caras
4004 Red Cedar Drive
Highlands Ranch, CO 80126

(303) 346-4949
www.DetoxifyYourLifestyle.com

Located in the heart of Highlands Ranch, CO - The leading health professionals at Premier Chiropractic and Natural Medicine are dedicated to helping you achieve your wellness objectives -- combining skill and expertise that spans the entire chiropractic wellness spectrum. Dr. Nick Caras is committed to bringing you optimal health and a better way of life by teaching and practicing the true principles of chiropractic wellness care.

Patients seeking treatment at Premier Chiropractic and Natural Medicine with Dr. Nick Caras are assured to receive only the finest quality care through the use of modern chiropractic equipment and technology. Dr. Nick Caras and the staff have a genuine concern for your well-being!

If you are interested in starting your journey towards wellness please subscribe to our award-winning newsletter at www.DetoxifyYourLifestyle.com. If you are already a newsletter subscriber, please explore the member wellness section of our website for wellness articles, resources, and health facts---specifically targeted by Dr. Nick Caras to your wellness needs and interests.

It's Your Life... Live it in Health!

Sex, Drugs & Rock N Roll
90-Day Companion Journal

The 90-Day Companion Journal supplements your commitment for creating a healthier lifestyle in an easy take-it-with-you journal.

Sex, Drugs & Rock N Roll is your new mantra for bringing more health and wellness to your family. Included are simple recipes, weekly menu planning, exercise goals and a place for your everyday thoughts and ideas. Look for it wherever *Sex, Drugs & Rock N Roll, 3 Keys To A Healthier Lifestyle* is sold.

Also by Dr. Nick Caras

Detoxify Your Lifestyle

Have you tried just about every diet on the menu, but continue to fight the battle of the bulge? Do you want to be free from sickness and disease, but still find yourself taking a cabinet full of medicine? Do you suffer depression, sleepless nights and know that there must be an answer to living a better life? It makes no difference what is prompting you to take control of your Life and live more naturally, if you want to detoxify your life, wellness guru Dr. Nick Caras wants to help. Dr. Caras offers clear directives on exercise, stress, fats, sugars and that when it comes to food - the greener the better! He wastes no time getting straight to the heart of the matter, which is your individual optimal fitness and well-being. Bold and straightforward, his health and wellness guide, *Detoxify Your*

182

Lifestyle puts the power where it should be - in your hands! A must read for taking your health and wellness to the next level and ensuring a great quality of life as you age! Your new lifestyle starts today.

"Detoxify Your Lifestyle" will teach you:

- The Secrets To Losing Weight The Right Way

- How To Boost Your Immune System

- Good Fats vs. Bad Fats

- The Truth About Sugars

- The Right Mindset

- Bacteria And Your Digestive Tract

- Good Exercise vs. Bad Exercise

- Nutrition And Your Kitchen

- Detoxifying Teammates

Also By Angel Tuccy

Lists That Saved My Life

As a perpetual list-maker and working mom, Angel Tuccy shares her secrets for balancing family, career and her personal life. This book will help you save time, save money and get more help from your family.

Lists That Saved My Business

This is the book that will revolutionize the way you do business. You have checklists to get everything done, but do you have lists to save your business? Using the database you already have, you can create a revolution in your own business.

Experience Pros Radio Show

The Experience Pros Radio Show is your daily in-your-pocket, in-the-car, in-your-office, business training. Live on AM 560 KLZ, Monday through Friday in Denver, CO.

Look up your local listings for times. Stream live at 560TheSource.com.

Participate in live chat and online conversation during the show at Facebook.com/ExperiencePros.

Download podcasts on iTunes or www.ExperiencePros.com

Instead Of

Instead of butter, try a light drizzle of olive oil.

Instead of creamy dressings, try a balsamic or oil & vinegar.

Instead of cheese dip, try salsa or hummus.

Instead of pastries, try a selection of bright berries.

Instead of topping with cheese, top with extra tomatoes.

Instead of boring celery sticks, try bell peppers in all the colors.

Instead of iceberg lettuce, try dark leafy lettuce greens.

Instead of pasta, add an extra serving of vegetables.

Instead of sweet tea or soda, try water with lemon.

Instead of salt, try new spices.

Instead of eating the "whole thing", try 3 bites.

Instead of stepping on the scale, let your clothes be your guide.

Instead of running long distances, try sprint intervals.

Instead of that bad habit, try replacing it with a healthy one.

Instead of complaining about what you can't have, be grateful

for your abundance.

About The Authors

Dr. Nick Caras is the best selling author of *Detoxify Your Lifestyle.* Dr. Nick has owned and operated two different Chiropractic and Natural Medicine clinics. Dr. Nick's current clinic is located in beautiful Highlands Ranch, CO, where he strives to stay on the cutting edge of the wellness revolution. The belief that health comes from within, not from outside sources like drugs and surgery is what keeps Dr. Caras motivated to help his patients. Dr. Nick and his wife, Heather, regularly travel the country to learn the latest techniques in natural medicine and how to treat almost any condition that will walk into his office. From the terminally ill, to patients who just want maintenance-wellness care, Dr. Nick strives to offer the best.

The Caras' reside in Highlands Ranch, CO and enjoy staying active while enjoying all that Colorado has to offer. In their off-time, they love traveling and Scuba diving throughout the Caribbean islands.

Angel Tuccy is the best selling author of *Lists That Saved My Life* and *Lists That Saved My Business*. Angel is a full-time working mom and entrepreneur. She is the founder of Experience Pros University and the host of a daily radio show in Denver, Colorado. She sits on the Board of Directors for the Chamber of Commerce of Highlands Ranch and she is a professional speaker for the South Metro Denver Chamber of Commerce. Angel runs the professional women's group "Ladies Who Lunch" and represents Ann Taylor clothing when she speaks.

Angel lives with her husband and three teenagers in beautiful Highlands Ranch, Colorado. She can be found on Facebook, search Experience Pros and at www.ExperiencePros.com.